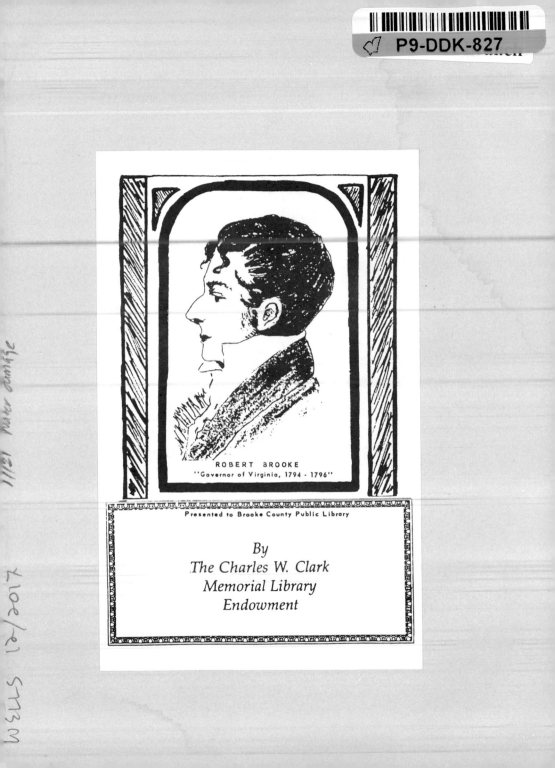

QUACKERY

A
BRIEF HISTORY
OF THE
WORST WAYS
TO CURE
EVERYTHING

LYDIA KANG, MD

NATE PEDERSEN

WORKMAN PUBLISHING · NEW YORK

·⊰ DEDICATION ⊱·

This one is for April for clearing the way. — NP

• • •

To my father and brother, two of the best
and most un-quacky physicians I know. And to my mother,
whose love can heal just about anything. — LK

Library of Congress Cataloging-in-Publication Data is available.

ISBN 978-0-7611-8981-7

Design by Janet Vicario

Workman books are available at special discounts when purchased in bulk for premiums and sales promotions as well as for fund-raising or educational use. Special editions or book excerpts can also be created to specification. For details, contact the Special Sales Director at the address below, or send an email to specialmarkets@workman.com.

Workman Publishing Company, Inc.
225 Varick Street
New York, NY 10014-4381
workman.com

WORKMAN is a registered trademark of Workman Publishing Co., Inc.

Printed in China
First printing October 2017

10 9 8 7 6 5 4 3 2 1

Contents

INTRODUCTION | v

ELEMENTS
Prescriptions from the Periodic Table

Mercury 3
Antimony 15
Arsenic 26
Gold 35
Radium & Radon 44

The Women's Health Hall of Shame 56

PLANTS & SOIL
Nature's Gifts

Opiates 61
Strychnine 72
Tobacco 83
Cocaine 95
Alcohol 105
Earth 115

The Antidotes Hall of Shame 124

TOOLS
Slicing, Dicing, Dousing, and Draining

Bloodletting 129
Lobotomy 140
Cautery & Blistering 151
Enemas & Clysters 163
Hydropathy & the
Cold Water Cure 173
Surgery 184

Anesthesia 195
The Men's Health Hall of Shame 206

ANIMALS
Creepy Crawlies, Corpses, and the Healing Power of the Human Body

Leeches 211
Cannibalism &
Corpse Medicine 221
Animal-Derived Medicines 233
Sex 244
Fasting 255

The Weight Loss Hall of Shame 266

MYSTERIOUS POWERS
Waves, Rays, and Curious Airs

Electricity 271
Animal Magnetism 281
Light 292
Radionics 303
The King's Touch 314

The Eye Care Hall of Shame 324
The Cancer Cure Hall of Shame 326

Acknowledgments 329
Index 332
Credits 343
About the Authors 344

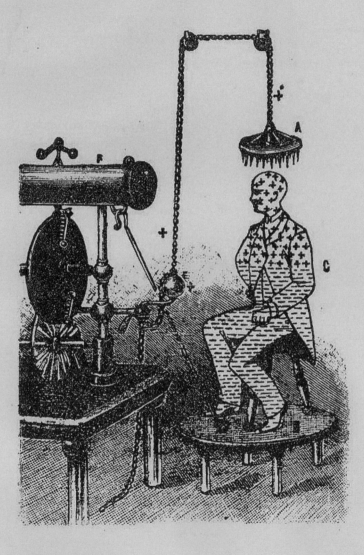

For shocks and giggles: a Russian electric shower.

Introduction

Humbug. Charlatan. Quack. Con artist. Swindler. Trickster.

For a long time, words like these were used to describe those who preyed on our fear of death and sickness by peddling wares that didn't work, or hurt us, or sometimes killed us.

But quackery isn't always about pure deception. Though the term is usually defined as the practice and promotion of intentionally fraudulent medical treatments, it also includes situations when people are touting what they truly believe works. Perhaps they're ignoring—or challenging—scientific fact. Or perhaps they lived centuries ago, before the scientific method entered civilization's consciousness. Through a modern-day lens, these treatments can seem absolutely absurd. Weasel nuts as a contraceptive? Bloodletting to help cure blood loss? Burning hot irons to fix the lovelorn? Yep.

But behind every misguided treatment—from Ottomans eating clay to keep the plague away to Victorian gents sitting in a mercury steam room for their syphilis to epilepsy sufferers sipping gladiator blood in ancient Rome—is the incredible power of the human desire to live. And this drive is downright inspiring: We are willing to ingest cadavers, subject ourselves to boiling oil, and endure experimental treatments involving way too many leeches, all in the name of survival.

This drive also leads to incredible innovation. After a long battle to achieve lower death rates (and reduce screaming), doctors now perform surgery when we're blissfully anesthetized. As an added bonus, their hands aren't dripping with pus from the prior surgery case. We can fight cancer on a molecular level, in ways our ancestors never dreamed. Diseases like syphilis and smallpox are no longer an enormous burden on society. It's easy to forget that along the way to this progress, innovators were scoffed at and shamed; patients suffered through their doctors' mistakes, and sometimes even died. None of today's medical achievements would have occurred without challenging the status quo.

But there is, of course, a dark side. That desire to heal and live longer is about as addictive as opium itself. Scientists, impersonating Icarus, try to best one another in making drugs more effective and more potent. Emperors send their alchemists on ridiculous quests to unlock immortality. Charlatans decide that you need a new pair of implanted goat testicles. Sometimes, we're so desperate for a cure, we'll reach for anything.

Even radioactive suppositories.

Let's be honest. Being healthy isn't enough for many of us. We want more—eternal youth, perfect beauty, boundless energy, the virility of Zeus. And herein the quack truly thrives. This is where we start to believe that arsenic wafers will give us that peaches-and-cream complexion and that elusive gold elixirs will fix broken hearts. Hindsight makes it easy to laugh at many of the treatments in this book, but no doubt Dr. Google has assisted you in searching for a simple cure to a pesky problem. None of us are immune to wanting a quick fix. A hundred years ago, you might have been the person buying that strychnine tonic!

Clearly, we needed to be saved from quacks—and from ourselves. The rise of patent medicines in the nineteenth century drove America to its turning point. With the Pure Food and Drug Act of 1906, the United States cracked down on false and misleading labels, unsafe ingredients in food, and the adulteration of medical and food products. In 1930, the watchdog bureau became known as the Food and Drug Administration (FDA). Later laws in 1938 covered medical devices and cosmetics, and a 1962 law added scientific rigor to the drug industry.

Did regulations cure America of its quackery? Of course not. Despite modern scientific breakthroughs, the FDA, and a pretty damn good under-standing of how the human body works, quackery's tentacles still touch almost every aspect of the healthcare and cosmetics industry. This is why you'll read a present-day update in many of our chapters. In a surprising twist, some quack cures, like leeches, have transformed into real, working treatments. But in many cases (like eating tapeworms for weight loss), quack-ery simply lingers on and on . . . and on.

To continue battling charlatans, we need a more complete understand-ing of how the human body functions and how disease works. We also need to keep open minds about ways to combat disease and improve longevity. Finally, we need to keep our guard up. There will always be quacks out there ready to take full advantage of human desperation before science and medi-cine can find solid solutions.

So how does one become a wary, discerning consumer with an open mind? Beware that quack medicine often relies on anecdotal evidence, or the endorsement of a celebrity physician, to convince us something works. Also, look deeper into claims made that "studies show XYZ is amazing." These "studies" should have been rigorously performed, peer-reviewed, and repeat-edly tested by various entities to show effectiveness. And they rarely are. Our own biases—confirmation bias, ingroup bias, postpurchase rationalization, and a host of others—all have heady effects on our ability to systematically evaluate treatments as varied as herbal cough drops, electronic cancer zap-pers, or pricey plasma-injected facials.

In the end, it comes down to a few simple questions. Do you believe there's solid evidence that it's going to work? Are you willing to risk the side effects? And we mustn't forget—how deep are your pockets?

After all, this book really is just a brief history of the worst ways to cure everything. No doubt, there are more "worst ways" yet to come.

AUTHORS' NOTE

This book is by no means an exhaustive encyclopedia of all treatments we now deem to be ridiculous—for that reason, you'll notice we focus mostly on past treatments rather than current ones. Furthermore, there were many topics we would have liked to cover in depth, but which we believe belong in their own book with a completely different tone, including religious-based medical quackery and the gross injustices of gay conversion therapy and racism-based treatments.

ELEMENTS

Prescriptions from the Periodic Table

Mercury

Of Roman Gods, Toilet Archeology, Drooling Syphilitics, an Immortal Wannabe, and Erroneous Snakes

The baby's hands and feet had become icy, swollen, and red. The flesh was splitting off, resembling blanched tomatoes whose skins peeled back from the fruit. She had lost weight, cried petulantly, and clawed at herself from the intense itching, tearing the raw skin open. Sometimes her fever reached 102 degrees.

"If she was an adult," her mother had noted, "she would have been considered to be insane, sitting up in her cot, banging her head with her hands, tearing out her hair, screaming, and viciously scratching anyone who came near."

Later on, her condition would be called *acrodynia*, or painful tips, named so for the sufferer's aching hands and feet. But in 1921, they called the baby's affliction Pink's Disease, and they were seeing more and more cases every year. For a while, physicians struggled to determine the etiology. It was blamed on arsenic, ergot, allergies, and viruses. But by the 1950s, the wealth of cases pointed to one common ingredient ingested by the sick kids—calomel.

Parents, hoping to ease the teething pain of their infants, rubbed one of many available calomel-containing teething powders into their babies' sore gums. Very popular at the time: Dr. Moffett's Teethina Powder, which also boasted that it "Strengthens the Child . . . Relieves the Bowel Troubles of Children of ANY AGE," and could, temptingly, "Make baby fat as a pig."

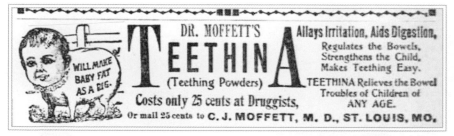

We, too, are freaked out by the baby-pig hybrid monster.

Beyond the creepy promise of Hansel and Gretel–esque results, there was something else sinister lurking within calomel: mercury. For hundreds of years, mercury-containing products claimed to heal a varied and strangely unrelated host of ailments. Melancholy, constipation, syphilis, influenza, parasites—you name it, and someone swore that mercury could fix it.

Mercury was used ubiquitously for centuries, at all levels of society, in its liquid

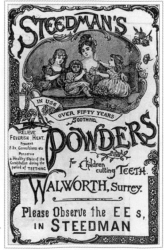

Spelling is everything if you're going to poison your kids correctly.

form (quicksilver) or as a salt. Calomel—also known as mercurous chloride—fell into the latter category and was used by some of the most illustrious personages in history, including Napoleon Bonaparte, Edgar Allan Poe, Andrew Jackson, and Louisa May Alcott. Why? That's a longer story.

CALOMEL: PURGING IT ALL AWAY

Drawing from the Greek words for *good* and *black* (named so for its habit of turning black in the presence of ammonia), calomel was *the* medicine from the sixteenth to the early twentieth century. Despite what it sounds like, calomel is nothing like caramel, though it sometimes carried the stomach-churning monikers "worm candy" and "worm chocolate" for treating parasites. By itself, calomel seems fairly innocuous—an odorless white powder. But don't be fooled: It's as harmless as your khaki-clad next-door neighbor who hides a basementful of bone saws. Taken orally, calomel is a potent cathartic, which is a sophisticated way of saying it will violently empty out your guts into the toilet. Constipation had long been associated with sickness, so opening the rectal gates of hell was a sign of righting the wrongs.

Some believe the "black" part of its name evolved from the dark stools ejected, which were mistaken for purged bile. Allowing bile to "flow freely" was in harmony with keeping the body balanced and the humors happy, a theory that harkened back to the time of Hippocrates and Galen. And if the insides of the bowels were dark and slimy, wasn't it better to rid the body of such toxins?

The "purging" occurred elsewhere, too—in the form of massive amounts of unattractive drooling, a symptom of mercury toxicity. A calomel consumer could give a rabid dog a run for its money. If the bad stuff was expelled via copious salivation, that was good, right? In the sixteenth century, Paracelsus believed that "effective" (i.e., toxic) doses of mercury were achieved when at least three pints of saliva were produced. That's a helluva lot of spit. And so, at a time when overflowing privies and gallons of loogie were the answer to a multitude of ailments, physicians found their drug of choice in calomel.

Benjamin Rush was one such physician. A founding father who signed the Declaration of Independence, Dr. Rush advocated for women's education and the abolition of slavery. He pioneered the humane treatment of psychiatric patients, but unfortunately thought that mental illness was best treated with a dose of calomel. He suggested this for the treatment of hypochondria:

> Mercury acts in this disease, 1, by abstracting morbid excitement from the brain to the mouth. 2, by removing visceral obstructions. And, 3, by changing the cause of our patient's complaints and fixing them wholly upon his sore mouth. The salivation will do still more service if it excite some degree of resentment against the patient's physician or friends.

Resentment against your doctor and BFF is a fantastic side effect! But in truth, Rush was replacing hypochondria with heavy metal toxicity. Another side effect was mercurial erethism, a neurological disorder that includes depression, anxiety, pathological shyness, and frequent sighing. Together with tremors of the limbs, these symptoms were often called mad hatter's disease or hatter's shakes (for the hat-making workers who used mercury in the felting process). In addition, toxic patients could suffer from lost teeth, rotting jaw bones, and gangrenous cheeks that produced facial holes, exposing ulcerated tongues and gums. Okay, so what if success

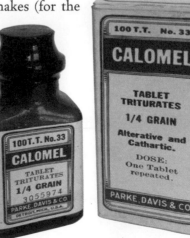

"Dose: One tablet repeated"
(until all hell breaks loose
in your toilet).

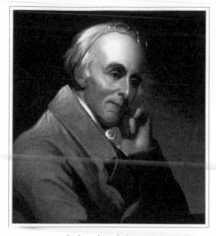

Benjamin Rush, founding father, wants you to poop excessively.

meant that Rush's patients turned into extremely moody *Walking Dead* extras?

When the mosquito-borne Yellow Fever virus hit Philadelphia in 1793, Dr. Rush became a passionate advocate of extreme amounts of calomel and bloodletting ("heroic depletion therapy"). Sometimes, ten times the usual calomel dose was employed. Even the purge-loving medical establishment found this excessive. Members of the Philadelphia College of Physicians called his methods "murderous" and "fit for a horse." Earlier, in 1788, author William Cobbett had labeled Rush a "potent quack."

At the time, Thomas Jefferson estimated the Yellow Fever fatality rate at 33 percent. Later, in 1960, the fatality rate of Rush's patients was found to be 46 percent. Not exactly an improvement on the status quo.

Ultimately, it was Dr. Rush's influence on improving Philadelphia's standing water problem and sanitation—plus a good, mosquito-killing first frost of autumn—that ended the epidemic. Alexander Hamilton, a friend of Dr. Rush, had become ill himself, but turned to another doctor who employed gentler methods. "In his theory of bleeding and mercury," Hamilton wrote, "I was ever opposed to my friend . . . whom I greatly loved; but who had done much harm, in the sincerest persuasion that he was preserving life." Hamilton survived, but Dr. Rush's reputation didn't. By the turn of the century, his medical practice dwindled to nothing.

Still, calomel continued to be used. It wasn't until the mid-twentieth century that mercury compounds finally fell out of favor, thanks to a solid understanding that heavy metal toxicity was actually, you know, *bad*.

QUICKSILVER: A BEASTLY BEAUTY

Most people know of elemental mercury as that slippery, silvery liquid once used with ubiquity in glass thermometers. If you were a child before helicopter parenting or organic anything, you might have had the opportunity to play with the contents of a broken thermometer. The glimmering balls skittered everywhere and delighted children for hours.

There was always something mystical about "quicksilver," as it was often called. Its older Latin name, *hydrargyrum*, spoke to its astonishing uniqueness—"water silver"—and gave rise to its Hg abbreviation on the periodic table of elements. The only metal that is liquid at room temperature, it's also the only element whose common name was taken from its association with alchemy and a Roman god.

So it almost makes sense that people expected magical things from mercury. Qin Shi Huang, First Emperor of the Qin Dynasty (246–221 BCE), was one of them. Desperate for the secret to immortality, he sent out search parties to find the answer, but they were doomed to fail. Instead, his own alchemists concocted mercury medicines, thinking that the shining liquid was the key.

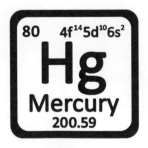

He died at the tender age of forty-nine from mercury poisoning. But hey, why stop there? In an attempt to rule in the afterlife, Qin had himself buried in an underground mausoleum so grand that ancient writers described it flowing with rivers of mercury, its ceiling decorated with jeweled constellations. It's also reportedly booby-trapped, Indiana Jones–style, with arrows that fire when disturbed. Happily for him and chillingly for everyone else, Qin made sure his concubines and tomb designers were buried alive right along with him. Brrr. Thus far, the tomb is unexcavated due to the toxic levels of mercury that threaten to release if it's opened.

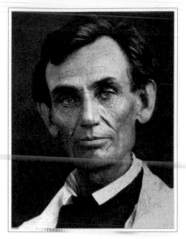

Abraham Lincoln, pre-beard, pre-hat, and not yet mercury-free.

Quite a bit later, when Abraham Lincoln was immortalizing himself in history, he too was a victim of liquid mercury. Before his presidency, Lincoln suffered from mood swings, headaches, and constipation. In the 1850s, an aide noted, "[W]hen he hed no passages he alwys had a sick headache—Took Blue pills—blue Mass." These "sick headaches" were also known as "bilious headaches" and could conceivably be cured by a good cathartic that also "allowed" bile to flow.

So what was this mysterious "blue mass"? A peppercorn-sized pill containing pure liquid mercury, licorice root, rosewater, honey, and sugar. Because liquid mercury is poorly absorbed in the intestine, druggists gleefully exercised their repressed aggressions by repeatedly pounding the liquid beads into relative oblivion, a process called extinction. Unfortunately, this violent compounding also allowed the mercury to be more readily absorbed in vapor form within the intestine.

Like a caffeine junkie guzzling down mislabeled decaf, Lincoln only grew worse after taking the pills. There are several accounts of his volatile behavior at the time, with bouts of depression mixed with rage, as well as insomnia, tremors, and gait problems, all of which could theoretically be blamed on mercury toxicity. He, too, may have suffered from erethism.

Lincoln, to his credit, seemed to recognize that the blue mass might be making him worse rather than better, and he apparently decreased his use once he entered the White House. And not a moment too soon. One shudders to imagine a mercury-toxic, pathologically moody leader of our nation calling the shots during the Civil War.

"A Night with Venus, a Lifetime with Mercury"

Mercury has had an entwined relationship with syphilis for centuries. In the fifteenth century after the French invasion of Naples, Italy, the disease began to make its way across Europe. As Voltaire noted, "On their flippant way through Italy, the French carelessly picked up Genoa, Naples, and syphilis. Then they were thrown out and deprived of Naples and Genoa. But they did not lose everything—syphilis went with them."

Soon, the "Great Pox" became a true nuisance and deadly accompaniment as it spread throughout Europe. That historical strain of *Treponema pallidum* (which is the responsible bacterium) was particularly virulent. Genital sores sprouted after exposure to an infected sexual partner and progressed to rash and fevers. Later, foul-smelling abscesses, pustules, and sores spread over the body, some so severe that they ate away at face, flesh, and bone. Yes. Out-of-control syphilis is pretty revolting.

People were desperate for a cure. By the sixteenth century, mercury came to the rescue with the help of the rather bombastic and vehement Paracelsus, who argued against Galen's humoral theory. He believed instead that mercury, salt, and sulfur would bring about all manner of bodily cures, having earth-bound, physiologic, and astrological qualities.

Another salt, mercuric chloride, arrived on the scene. Unlike calomel, mercuric chloride was water-soluble and easily absorbed by the body, making its poisonous results seem all the more effective. It burned the skin when applied ("It hurts! Therefore, it works!"), and the copious salivation was considered a sign of successful purging.

Syphilitic patients also received what sound like the worst spa packages ever. Elemental mercury was heated for steam baths, where inhalation was considered beneficial (and is a potent route of mercury absorption). Mercuric chloride was added to fat, and the resultant unction rubbed dutifully into

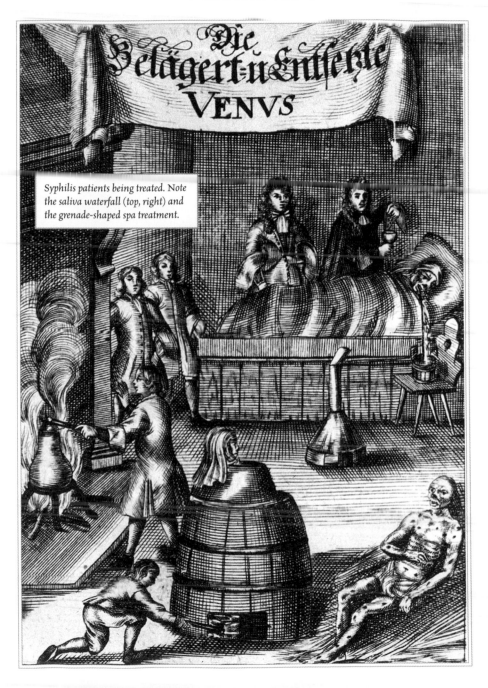

Die Belägert-u. Entsetzte VENVS

Syphilis patients being treated. Note the saliva waterfall (top, right) and the grenade-shaped spa treatment.

LEWIS AND CLARK AND THE THUNDERBOLTS
(NO, IT'S NOT A BAND)

Benjamin Rush's influence had more far-reaching effects beyond Philadelphia, in the form of Dr. Rush's Bilious Pills. The pills, a proprietary blend of calomel, chlorine, and jalap (a potent herbal laxative), were fondly referred to as Dr. Rush's Thunderbolts or "Thunderclappers." On Rush's recommendations, Lewis and Clark took them on their famous expedition. Rush wrote, "When you feel the least indisposition . . . gently open the bowels by means of one, two, or more of the purging pills." Also, constipation "is often a sign of approaching disease . . . take one or more of the purging pills." In addition, lack of appetite "is a sign of approaching indisposition and it should be obviated by the same remedy."

In summary, if anything felt off? Purge. Purge like hell.

So Lewis and Clark brought no less than 600 of Dr. Rush's Thunderbolts. Modern historians determined that on their historic

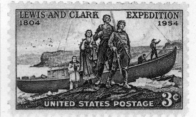

To boldly purge where no man has purged before.

journey, Lewis and Clark had squatted in Lolo, Montana—literally. As their expedition was a military one, they relied on military guidelines that ordered their latrines be located 300 feet from the main camping area, which had been found using dated lead samples. Lo and behold, mercury was detected 300 feet away. It was an excremental bingo winner. Rush's Thunderbolts may or may not have cured their ills, but they certainly left their mark, in a scatalogically historical way.

sores. Sometimes, bodily fumigations occurred, where a naked patient was placed in a box with some liquid mercury, their head sticking out of a hole, and a fire lit beneath the box to vaporize the mercury. Sixteenth-century Italian physician Girolamo Fracastoro remarked that after mercury ointments and fumigations, "You will feel the ferments of the disease dissolve themselves in your mouth in a disgusting flow of saliva."

Treatment for syphilis was vastly unsexy. What was worse, these regimens would often continue for the rest of the sufferer's life. There was no denying a common saying at the time: "A night with Venus, and a lifetime with mercury."

Niccolò Paganini, one of the most famous violinists in history, likely suffered from mercury toxicity after he was diagnosed with syphilis. Besides suffering from hypochondria and excessive shyness from erethism, he also began shaking uncontrollably, contributing to his withdrawal from the stage in 1834. He had tree-trunk legs and coughed gunk up chronically. He complained, "I easily expectorate the mucus and pus . . . three or four saucerfuls . . . the swelling in my legs has risen to behind the knees so that I walk like a snail." His teeth fell out, his bladder was constantly irritated, and his testicles became inflamed to the size of "a little pumpkin." Damn you, syphilis, for ruining the adorableness of little pumpkins everywhere.

Luckily, or unluckily, poor Paganini's horrid life of mucus production, mollusk-like speed, and gourd-sized nether regions didn't last long. Within a month after he stopped performing, Paganini was dead.

Nowadays, we do know that mercury and other metals such as silver can kill bacteria in vitro. All scientists know, however, that what's good in the petri dish isn't necessarily good in the human body. It's unclear if syphilis sufferers were cured by their mercury treatments or if they simply moved on to the next phase of the illness, which could consist of many symptom-free years.

That is, if the mercury toxicity didn't kill them first.

THE CADUCEUS: A SNAKE SWITCHEROO

Calomel fell from favor gradually, as safer and more effective treatments replaced the "heroic medicine" of purging. In the United States and around the world, mercury was banned from felting in the 1940s and gold and silver mining in the 1960s. Calomel wasn't removed from the British pharmacopoeia until the 1950s because it took that long to finally realize mercury was the cause of acrodynia. Even now, you can still find mercury thermometers (they're more accurate than the red-colored alcohol ones), but regulations are phasing them out worldwide.

Though the element is no longer used in mainstream medicine, mercury has managed to slither its way into many a doctor's office. It is perhaps oddly appropriate that the symbol for the god Mercury was the caduceus—two snakes entwined on a winged rod. The symbol is commonly and incorrectly associated with the medical establishment, due to a mistake when the US Army Medical Corps adopted the symbol in 1902. Soon after, it became a ubiquitous sign of healing. But in fact, the caduceus represents Mercury—the god of financial gain, commerce, thieves, and trickery.

The Rod of Asclepius, which has a single serpent entwined on a simple rod, was held by the Greek god Asclepius, the patron of health and healing. This was the rod mistakenly missed in 1902 and is currently used by most academic medical establishments today.

In 1932, Stuart Tyson argued about the misuse of the caduceus in *The Scientific Monthly*, stating that Mercury was "the patron of commerce and of the fat purse . . . his silver tongued eloquence could always make 'the worse appear the better cause.' . . . Would not his symbol be suitable for . . . all medical quacks?" Indeed.

Mercury, holding his caduceus and a fat purse, while stomping on everyone.

2

JAMES'S FEVER ~
~ J. L. RIDDLE, CHE~
~ LATE OF
31 HUNTER STREET, BRUNSW~
LONDON.

Sold in BOTTLES containing ONE OU~
PACKETS at 2s. 6d. ea~

~essrs. BARCLAY & ~ons, ~ndon, 95 Farrin~
have been appointed Sole Wholesale A~
January, 1878.

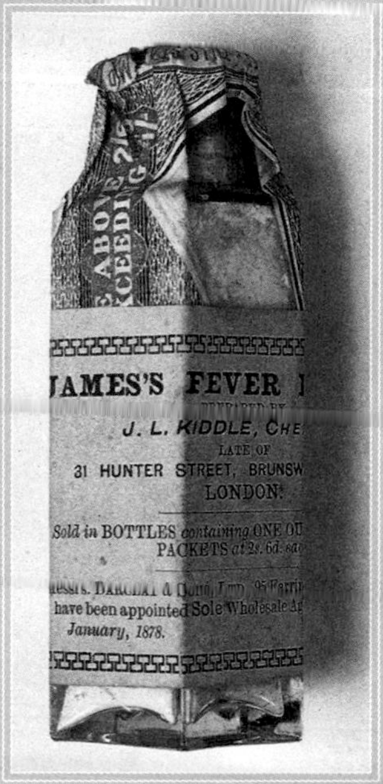

Antimony

Of Oliver Goldsmith's Last Folly,
the Fake Basil Valentine, Captain Cook's Cup,
and Everlasting Poop Pills

In 1774, **Oliver Goldsmith** was feeling rather off. The forty-four-year-old author of *The Vicar of Wakefield* and *She Stoops to Conquer* had a fever, headache, and suspected kidney problems. In his life, he'd graduated at the bottom of his class at Trinity College, attempted but did not complete a degree in medicine in Edinburgh, and wandered Europe after exhausting his funds. He finally managed a degree of success as a writer, though some, like Horace Walpole, called him "an inspired idiot."

It was, however, his incomplete doctorate in medicine and briefly held position as an apothecary's assistant that led to action at that moment. He must cure himself.

It was time for St. James's Fever Powder.

Now, St. James's Fever Powder was famous in its time. Created and sold by one of the eighteenth century's most famous patent medicine doctors, the powder claimed to cure fevers "accompanied by convulsions and light-headedness," gout,

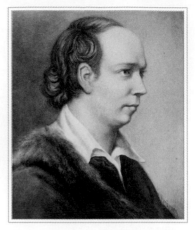

Oliver Goldsmith, author and "inspired idiot."

scurvy, and cattle distemper virus. Dr. Robert James was so secretive about his formula that he even lied on his patent application for fear others would steal it. But the main ingredient, a toxic metal called antimony, was extremely good at what Oliver Goldsmith thought he needed—nay, demanded—to get him out of his sickbed.

He wanted to vomit.

Goldsmith, who called himself a doctor despite not being one, asked an apothecary to bring him St. James's Fever Powder. The apothecary resisted, begging him to consult a real physician. But Goldsmith ended up getting what he asked for.

Eighteen hours later, after a lot of vomiting and convulsions, Oliver Goldsmith was dead.

A Brief History of Hurling

We'll get back to poor Mr. Goldsmith and his coveted antimony prescription. But first, let's take a brief pause to examine why he wanted to vomit so badly that it killed him.

Emesis, or vomiting, is the body's way of ridding itself of its stomach contents, against both gravity and the body's normal digestional direction. By irritating the lining of the stomach, eliciting the gag reflex, and tickling the "vomiting center" in your brain (yes, that's a real neural location), you can induce this reverse digestion. Emetics like antimony are substances you take on purpose to make you spew, and they have a long and glorious history. Herodotus reported that the ancient Egyptians employed monthly emetics to maintain their health. Hippocrates, too, advocated regular vomiting. The recommendations go on and on through several millennia. Up until only a few decades ago, emetics were still considered an important part of the medical formulary.

Much of emetics' use linked back to humoral theories of the body: It was believed that when the body's blood, black bile, yellow bile, or phlegm was unbalanced, sickness occurred. So rebalancing via vomiting, diarrhea, sweating, or salivation was necessary. Basically, if it could ooze out of a pore or projectile shoot out of an orifice, it *balanced* you.

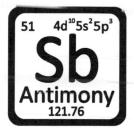

And since 3000 BCE, antimony, a grayish metalloid mined from mineral deposits around the world, was the substance du jour for this purpose. It's well known that some people have enjoyed emetics for their ability to empty themselves out after a gluttonous meal, as Roman emperors Julius Caesar and Claudius were known to do. Seneca the Younger, counsel to Emperor Nero, mentioned some Romans who "vomited to eat, and ate to vomit, and did not deign to digest their repasts furnished from all parts of the world." An antimony-containing wine was reportedly used for such purposes. (Interestingly, the term *vomitorium* was long thought to be an area provided to bingeing Roman partygoers. But in actuality, it was simply an exit area of an amphitheater for crowds to "purge" and leave the building. That's right. It's an architectural term that equates people with vomit.)

Unfortunately, to get the body to reverse its normal processes, sometimes you have to introduce it to something it desperately wants to remove, like poison. Scholars and healers alike recognized antimony's toxic potential. It could cause liver damage, severe inflammation of the pancreas, heart problems, and death. Still, they were confident that doctors could rein in its lethal power. A common thought at the time regarding antimony was that "a poison is not a poison in the hands of a physician."

Too bad that Oliver Goldsmith got his antimony, despite his doctors' disagreement.

MONK KILLER OR WONDER DRUG?

Sixteenth-century celebrity physician Paracelsus believed in a more mineral-based philosophy as opposed to humors, a radical divergence of thought that brought him plenty of followers and enemies. One must understand the natural sciences before understanding the body's ailments, he believed. Earthly substances like antimony or mercury were the perfect elements to set things right. Antimony in particular "purifies itself and at the same time everything else that is impure," he claimed.

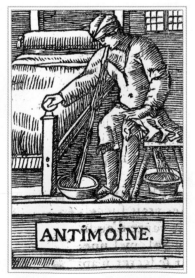

You'd think the endorsement of the Renaissance's Dr. Oz would be enough to make you the go-to vomit inducer, but it wasn't until antimony received a mythical monk's stamp of approval that it really took off.

Antimony's name supposedly draws from a story about a fifteenth-century German monk named Basil Valentine.

He's got good aim, doesn't he?

Legend has it, he belonged to the Canon of Benedictine Priory of St. Peter and died at an astounding 106 years old. His mysterious epitaph read: "*post CXX annos patebo*" (after 120 years to clear, or, perhaps, pass), and right on the mark, one of the priory's church pillars reportedly burst open to reveal hidden books written by Valentine, the existence of which no one ever knew.

Valentine extolled the virtues of antimony in a manuscript entitled "The Triumphant Chariot of Antimony." He even recommended it to fatten up pigs. Rumor told that after having a good effect on the swine, he tried it on monks, who promptly died. Hence the meaning of *antimony*—"anti-monk" or "monk killer." (This is unlikely the true origin. Antimony more likely derives from the Greek word *antimonos*, for "a metal not found alone," due to its natural affinity for other elements like sulfur. Just as "Basil Valentine" is more apt a name for a sleazy lounge singer.)

Valentine's manuscripts had magically entered the hands of one Johann Thölde, a salt boiler, salesman, and the likely true author of the texts. He also happened to be a skilled chemist. In the early 1600s, he made a pretty penny spreading Valentine's writing around, and antimony experienced a surge in use.

And an intellectual war began.

Galenical physicians who extolled the virtues of humoral theory were in a rage about the doctor-chemists who followed Paracelsus and Valentine and adored the purgative powers of mercury and antimony. Bitter fights and court battles ensued over the intersection of chemistry and medicine, with antimony at their center. The faculty of medicine in Paris decreed antimony was a "virulent poison." One of the loudest seventeenth-century French critics, physician Guy Patin, exclaimed, "May God protect us from such drugs and such physicians!"

And yet, many believed antimony would "perfect the body" and would purify anything impure it came to touch. It was used for everything from asthma and allergies to syphilis and the plague. When King Louix XIV fell deathly ill in 1658, he received a dose. He recovered (miraculously), and that ended the antimony debate in France with one shiny, metalloid winner.

And what of Thölde and the possibly fictitious Valentine? No one really cared that the salt boiler/chemist was likely the true author of the texts. It seemed quite impossible that a fifteenth-century monk would have written the manuscript because "Valentine" referenced things that happened *after* his death. But the nauseating legacy of antimony was very real indeed.

Everlasting Pills and Puke Chalices

At the height of antimony's popularity, it wasn't enough to pop the occasional prescription. People had to possess *accessories*. Fashionable in the seventeenth and eighteenth centuries, cups were made out of antimony, fondly called *pucula emetic* or *calicos vomitorii*—basically some version of "puke chalice." Combined with the acid in wine, the antimony from the cup would form "tartar emetic"—antimony potassium tartrate—and treat the cup holder to a good "healthy" vomit, or at least some diarrhea. One of the only remaining antimony cups is believed to have belonged to Captain James Cook, who may have taken it on his voyages around the world. But it wasn't to be used lightly—if too much antimony leached into the wine, the resulting drink would be deadly. One such cup, purchased in London's Gunpowder Alley in 1637 for 50 shillings, killed three people.

Then there were antimony pills. Unlike our one-use pharmaceuticals today, these metal pills were heavy, and after passing through the

To boot 'n' rally, just add wine: antimony cup and case, seventeenth century.

bowels they were often relatively unchanged. They were dutifully retrieved from latrines, washed, and reused over and over again. Talk about recycling. The "everlasting pills" or "perpetual pills" were often lovingly handed down from generation to generation as an heirloom. Imagine reading that in someone's last will and testament: "And to Jonathan, my beloved constipated son, I bequeath my poop pills."

And you thought Willy Wonka's Everlasting Gobstopper was special.

Plenty of enterprising quack doctors got rich off the antimony craze. After curing King George II of a dislocated thumb, eighteenth-century physician Joshua Ward could do no wrong in the king's eyes. Even though he had no medical background and a trifling knowledge of pharmaceuticals, Ward used his fame to amass a fortune. His signature medicines? Ward's Pill and Ward's Drop, which he claimed could cure every single human malady from gout to cancer. Too good to be true? Well, yes. They contained poisonous amounts of antimony. But everyone wanted Ward's Pill and Drop in their cupboards. Ever the promotional whiz, he even colored the pills red, purple, or blue because artificial color makes everything better, like Jell-O. Unlike Jell-O, some of Ward's formulations also contained arsenic. Ward did use his fortune to try and give back, even opening his own hospital. He ministered to the poor, which was quite good of him. Though he often gave them his pills—not so good of him.

THE HEALING POWER OF PAIN:
BLISTERING & AVERSION THERAPY

Given antimony's disgusting reputation, it might come as a surprise that people also used it on their faces. That's right. The same metal that caused emperors to spew and was used in everlasting poop pills was once employed as a cosmetic. Its abbreviation on the periodic table of elements, *Sb*, derives from stibnite, the sulfide mineral form of antimony. A light metallic gray that turns black when

A GAG-INDUCING POTPOURRI

Emetics come in a range of forms, typically mineral or herbal. Here's a rundown of some of history's most infamous puke-enhancers.

Salt Ancient mariners knew that drinking seawater could cause a good upchuck. The Greeks used a combination of salt, water, and vinegar. Pliny the Elder recommended a nice mixture of honey, rainwater, and seawater called *thalassomeli* to do the trick. Celsus described using wine and seawater, or salted Greek wine, to "loosen the belly," which is the gentlest way ever to say vomit. Of course, drinking heavily salted water can make you vomit, but it can also kill you.

Beer and crushed garlic Philumenus, a Greek physician from the fourth century, thought that a combination of beer and crushed garlic could cure poisonous asp bites via vomiting. Given that snakebite poison doesn't collect in the stomach, seems like you're adding insult to injury here.

Blue vitriol (copper sulfate) A crystalline substance with a striking blue color, it's been used as an emetic since the ninth century. In an 1839 magazine, blue vitriol is recommended for opium and hemlock poisonings. Unfortunately, blue vitriol is itself poisonous: It causes red blood cells to pop, muscle tissues to break down, and kidneys to fail.

Ipecac (short for ipecacuanha) First brought to Europe in the 1600s. No, it's not mentioned in a song called "The Girl from Ipecacuanha." Syrup of ipecac was used for centuries as an expectorant and emetic. For years, ipecac was also used for poisoning and was considered a necessary component of every parent's medicine cabinet in the nineteenth and early twentieth centuries. It's still available today. But modern toxicologists know it doesn't reliably decrease the absorption of toxins, and half the time, it doesn't even make you throw up. And the song is "The Girl from Ipanema," okay?

Apomorphine This hallucinogenic drug comes from the bulbs and roots of certain water lilies (the *Nymphaea* genus). Used by the Maya and immortalized on ancient Egyptian tomb frescoes, the drug was eventually synthesized in the mid-1800s. And it was potent. A 1971 review described its success rate as nearly perfect in ensuring vomiting, compared to the 30 to 50 percent rate of other emetics. It was unfortunately once used in homosexual aversion therapy, and even killed some of its "patients." It is now used, carefully, in veterinary medicine, and, rarely, for human Parkinson's disease.

Pretty blue copper sulfate. Looks like rock candy. Do not lick.

exposed to air, stibnite was used around the eyes in ancient Egypt, the Middle East, and parts of Asia (where it is known as *kohl*).

But before you reach for some stibnite to give yourself a smoky eye, read on. If you thought antimony could do a number on your guts, just wait till you hear what it can do to your skin. In the realm of counterirritation—the theory that burning or blistering one part of the body would draw illness away from a sick area (see Cautery & Blistering, page 151)—antimony was also used topically as a blistering agent. An 1832 London medical encyclopedia recommends an antimony-based ointment to cure whooping cough and tuberculosis. Which, for the record, it can't. Oh, and that blister it created? Apparently, the encyclopedia's authors thought it would be better to keep it alive forever. Meaning, when the blister was starting to heal, you'd rip the top off and add more tartar emetic in order to "yield a copious secretion of pus."

Gross. Who says topical antimony can't also make you throw up?

Antimony advocates took this no-pain, no-gain approach even further with aversion therapy, a behavior treatment that works to associate something you want (like drinking alcohol) with something you hate (like puking up your guts). Philadelphia physician Benjamin Rush once slipped a few grains of tartar emetic into a glass of rum for a man who loved the liquor a little too much. After vomiting, the patient had an aversion to the drink for two years, much to Rush's delight. So, one might think antimony would be great for this purpose except, oops, it's really freaking toxic, and alcoholism isn't a disease with a quick fix.

And yet, quacks persisted. In 1941, a court case arose alleging that Mrs. Moffat's Shoo-Fly Powders for Drunkenness, which contained antimony, were fraudulent and toxic (not to mention that the name was sort of ridiculous). But that didn't stop people from continuing to use it for alcoholism. In fact, antimony is still used outside of the United States for this purpose. In 2004, a nineteen-year-old man drank Guatemalan "Soluto Vital," an antimony-based beverage that damaged his kidneys. The *New England Journal of Medicine* highlighted a 2012 case of a man who went home drunk and received a dose of *tártaro emético* from his wife. She had purchased it in Central America, after being told it would cause vomiting and make him stop drinking alcohol. He too landed in the hospital with kidney and liver damage.

These days, there are still sanctioned medicines for aversion therapy, like Antabuse, a chemical that makes you vomit in the presence of ingested alcohol. And yet, it's not commonly used because, surprise! Patients don't like to take it. Ah, aversion to aversion therapy. And it doesn't even involve antimony.

PURGING ANTIMONY FROM OUR SYSTEMS

There's a reason why there are no medicines in the modern pharmacopeia that purposely induce vomiting, aside from Antabuse. We have better ways of handling ingested poison. Nowadays, activated charcoal is given to adsorb toxins in the stomach, and chelation therapies can bind them up in the blood. No upchucking necessary!

Antimony may have been a miraculous substance to followers of Paracelsus and Valentine, but burning blisters and puke chalices aren't all that appreciated today. Though it's used in some countries to treat certain parasitic infections, in the United States it's not approved. Antimony compounds have a lot of side effects similar to arsenic, such as sore mouth, kidney failure, and of course, nausea, vomiting, and abdominal pain. And there's this other little problem—it's also carcinogenic.

Too bad Oliver Goldsmith didn't know all this before he got what he asked for.

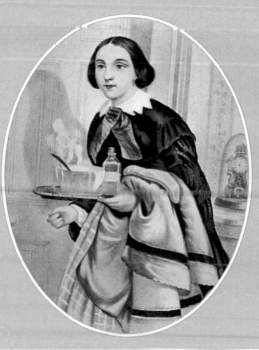

3

Arsenic

Of Inheritance Powder, Ratsbane Eaters, the Hot Milkmaid Who Died to Be Pretty, the Savior of Syphilis, and Poisonous Wallpaper

Meet Mary Frances Creighton—a wife, sister, and mother with a talent for getting away with murder. The first time she killed, the victim was her mother-in-law in 1920. People thought the wealthy forty-seven-year-old woman died of ptomaine poisoning. But Mary had fed her some toothsome hot cocoa just before she began to violently vomit. She was dead within hours.

In 1923, Mary struck again. She'd persuaded her teenage brother, Charles, to move in with her and her husband, even feeding him chocolate pudding

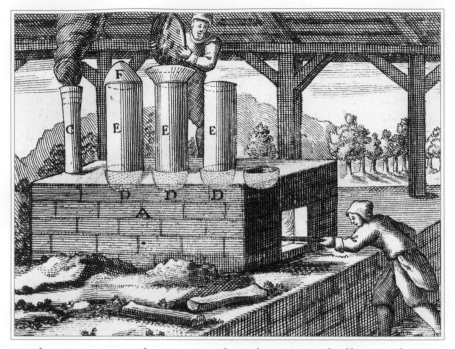

Manufacturing arsenic, 1704. A favorite among murderers, white arsenic is produced by roasting the arsenic sulfide mineral.

before bedtime. Charles fell sick with stomachaches and a dry mouth. He died a rather horrible death soon after, stricken with vomiting and shaking.

It was blamed on a bad stomach virus. But how convenient that Mary had just become a beneficiary in a $1,000 life insurance policy for Charles. The police were alerted via an anonymous letter that Mary Frances was a liar, and the boy, a victim. Bodies were exhumed, and forensic chemists tested the bodies of both Charles and Mary's mother-in-law. The answer? Arsenic.

Better known for its ability to kill than heal, arsenic is a potent liver toxin and a carcinogen. A lethal dose (around 100 mg) will usually render the victim dead within several hours. From the Middle Ages until the turn of the twentieth century, arsenic was fondly known as "the king of poisons," "the poison of kings," and "inheritance powder." Even Hippocrates knew of its toxicity in

ancient times, describing a type of abdominal colic seen in miners who uncov
ered arsenic. Roman Emperor Nero found these effects to be quite handy,
using arsenic to kill off his brother Britannicus and ensure his own title.

Why was arsenic the go-to poison for everyone, from housewives to
emperors? For starters, it's virtually undetectable. Its most famous form,
"white arsenic," is odorless and, when concealed in food and drink, often
tasteless. The symptoms are also helpfully similar to food poisoning. In times
before refrigeration, when a king suddenly started having stomach cramps,
vomiting his brains out, and filling the chamber pots with diarrhea, it wasn't
always obvious a killer was at hand. The Medici and Borgia families in renaissance Europe used arsenic generously to kill off whomever got in their way.
English essayist Max Beerbohm once said, "No Roman ever was able to say, 'I
dined last night with the Borgias.'"

And even though Mary Frances Creighton earned nicknames like "the
Long Island Borgia," she was found not guilty of either suspicious death. In
fact, she would go on to poison yet
another person with arsenic years
later. (Well, why not? It worked great
the first two times!) In that case, it
was Ada Appelgate, the wife of the
man who was having an affair with
Mary's teenage daughter.

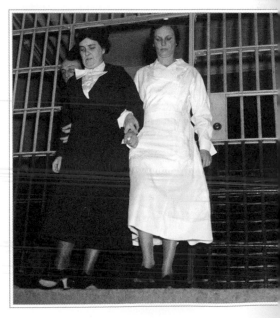

Although it seemed like an
open-and-shut case, there was a key
reason Mary's crime was so difficult
to prove: In the early twentieth century, arsenic was everywhere.

Mary Frances Creighton, the "Long Island Borgia,"
heads to court, 1936.

Take Two Arsenic and
Don't Call Me in the Morning

Arsenic has been used since antiquity as a medicinal. It's an escharotic, which means it causes the skin surface to die and slough off. So in conditions where the skin is abnormally thickened, like psoriasis, it worked, but it was applied to *all* skin problems, including ulcers or eczema. A dab here or there might not do too much harm, but excessive or extended use can cause chronic arsenic toxicity. And like many medicinals in history, arsenic was used for a hell of a lot that didn't make sense: fevers, stomach pain, heartburn, rheumatism, and as a general tonic. From Aiken's Tonic Pills to Compound Sulphur Lozenges to Gross's Neuralgia Pills, the quackery-laden patent medicine trade was loving arsenic in the eighteenth century.

Also on the market: arsenic-based antimalarials like Tasteless Ague and Fever Drops (a selling point because the alternative, quinine, was bitter). Did they kill the malaria parasite? It's unclear. But some doctors scathingly noted that arsenic could "heal fevers by killing patients." A doctor named Thomas Fowler thought it helped, and he went about making his own formula that would reign as the best-known arsenical medicine for 150 years.

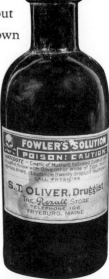

Fowler's Solution, created in 1786, was 1 percent potassium arsenate with lavender flavoring added to prevent it from being accidentally mistaken for water. There were claims that it cured syphilis, a parasitic infection known as sleeping sickness, and fevers due to *remitting ague*, a term for malaria. Since doctors knew it could burn away some skin disorders, they applied it to cancerous tumors in the hope of dissolving them. An 1818 dispensatory details the disappointing results: "unfortunately its

Note that half the label is filled with poison warnings and antidotes.

good effects often do not go beyond a certain length," and for many patients, "it must be allowed it does harm." It could cause a thiamine deficiency, leaving people with tingling extremities and racing hearts.

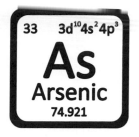

33   $3d^{10}4s^24p^3$
As
Arsenic
74.921

As a health tonic to boost vitality, Fowler's was all show and no substance. The arsenic had a tendency to dilate small capillaries in the face. So people got flushed cheeks and a look of bloom and health—but they didn't actually feel better. And as with many other medicinals like mercury, arsenic toxicity could cause some alarming symptoms, including diarrhea or confusion. It had an effect on the body, which in a time before modern lab tests and scans, was one of the ways that people knew a medicine was doing *something* (if excessive flatulence counts).

Aside from Fowler's Solution, arsenic products continued to be used freely throughout much of the nineteenth century. They were applied to the skin, used in enemas, and eaten. One favorite way to consume it was by adding it to bread and making "bread pills," or with pepper. It was also injected and inhaled in vapor form. One pharmacology textbook touted arsenic as being safe to give to nursing mothers, who could treat their babies via arsenic-laden breastmilk. Others used it for morning sickness. The diseases it was claimed to heal were endless. Snakebites! Rickets! Drunken vomiting! All of it could be cured with arsenic. Or so people believed.

Fowler's Solution and arsenicals were, however, still recognized as "capricious, unpredictable and uncontrollable both as to good and harm," according to a 1948 pharmacology text by Torald Sollmann. Karl Marx reportedly stopped using it because it "dulls my mind too much." Charles Darwin was believed to suffer from arsenic poisoning due to his use of Fowler's. Over time, arsenic thickens and darkens the skin, and his bronzed appearance, no matter how little sun exposure he'd gotten, pointed to this possibility. One Jonathan Hutchinson revealed that arsenic's effect "is not to give vigor but to diminish it, and make the patient feel apathetic and uncomfortable." Patients begged him, "Please don't order me arsenic, for it always makes me feel so ill."

Another person who had a bottle of Fowler's on her shelf? Mary Frances Creighton. But it would have taken gallons of the diluted solution to reach the levels of arsenic found in Charles's body—not exactly easy to blend into a few servings of pudding. So how did Charles get such a ridiculous amount of poison in his body?

Perhaps, Mary's lawyers suggested, he was ingesting arsenic on purpose. Sound crazy? Then you haven't met the toxiphagi.

The Arsenic Eaters of Styria

The toxiphagi were a group of villagers in Styria, an area that is now part of Austria, who ate arsenic on purpose. A lot of it. They were also known as ratsbane eaters (so called because arsenic was a great rodenticide—it was in the Rough on Rats poison that Mary Creighton used on her brother and Ada Appelgate, the public would soon learn). A Swiss physician, Johann Jakob von Tschudi, first reported on the toxiphagi in 1851. Apparently, these villagers would consume small amounts of arsenic, perhaps one-half grain (about 30 milligrams) a few times a week, building up to lethal doses of up to eight grains (about 500 milligrams). The chunks of white arsenic resembled chalk and were sprinkled on bread or "on a small lump of fresh lard." Yummy. It was purchased from "wandering herbalists or peddlers, who, on their part, obtain[ed] it from workmen in Hungarian glass, from veterinary surgeons, and from charlatans." Not exactly Pfizer, but okay.

Styrians boasted of increased endurance and sexual appetite, blooming cheeks, and robustness in the form of weight gain. (They even gave arsenic to their horses.) Tschudi reported of a milkmaid who wanted to increase her charms to attract a certain lover. She started taking arsenic and "after a few months she became plump, chubby, in a word all that the swain would desire." She figured, well, why stop there? The milkmaid increased her dosage until she "fell victim to her coquetry. She died poisoned, and her end was a painful one." Unfortunately, the theory that "more is better" is a really, really crappy theory when it comes to arsenic.

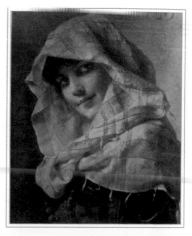

A Styrian peasant girl, circa 1898. A face that sold a lot of poison.

Oddly enough, the toxiphagi seemed to become addicted to their chosen poison. If they stopped taking it, they'd suffer the effects of withdrawal, including appetite loss, anxiety, vomiting, excessive salivation, constipation, and breathing problems. Death occurred, too, unless the toxiphagi resumed their diet. What's more, the arsenic eaters didn't all glow with a healthy bloom—many died hideous deaths.

At the time, news of the toxiphagi shook the medical community around the world. In the *Boston Medical and Surgical Journal* (the forerunner to the *New England Journal of Medicine*), a Dr. Chevallier proclaimed, "The facts reported have appeared to us so improbably, that we have put no faith in them." It was thought that some of the arsenic being eaten was actually chalk, sold by charlatans. Others believed that the chunky doses of arsenic were not fully absorbed. Eventually, other physicians reported real arsenic in many of the toxiphagi's diets, although without a modern blood analysis, the arsenic-eater story is still hard to swallow.

No matter how one interprets their story, it's indisputable that reports of the toxiphagi transformed arsenic's reputation from feared poison to youth-restorer and cure-all. Sadly, the idea of a beautiful arsenic eater made its mark on society. There were plenty of ladies willing to eat poison and unwillingly die for beauty.

PRETTY AND DEAD = PRETTY DEAD:
ARSENIC THE COSMETIC

The story of the milkmaid from Styria spread through Europe, where others sought to become blushing beauties (ignoring, perhaps, her inconvenient death). In the Victorian era, a cocktail of arsenic, vinegar, and chalk could cause anemia, which in turn made the skin appear paler and more aristocratic. As mentioned earlier, arsenic dilates capillaries, giving some a flush of health. But in reality, chronic absorption actually darkens one's complexion, so likely the side ingredients or other efforts (staying out of the sun or using vinegar washes) did more than the poison to pale the skin. Thankfully, plenty of cosmetic products didn't have large doses of arsenic. If they did? A smart consumer might stop using the product once the opposite effect was noticed.

Still, the arsenic cosmetic fad persisted. In the nineteenth century, drinking or rinsing one's face with Fowler's Solution and using arsenical supplements and soaps was quite fashionable. There were even hair tonics that boasted arsenic in their contents, never mind that it actually causes hair loss and has been used as a depilatory since the time of Hippocrates.

Scoring a point for logic, many decried the fashion. "What prospect is this for the man whose wife is thus absurdly immolating herself on the altar of vanity!" wrote one physician in 1878. A textbook case: Kate Brewington Bennett. She was reportedly the most beautiful woman in St. Louis and renowned for her porcelain-white skin. After consuming arsenic for years, she died at the age of thirty-seven, in 1855. Vain until the end, the beautiful lady begged her husband not to put her birthdate on her graveyard monument, so she would be immortalized as youthful. Her husband agreed, but sneakily added her age anyway.

Somewhere in the next life, the Bennetts are having a little lover's quarrel over that.

DON'T LICK THE WALLPAPER

Arsenic also made a beautiful array of dyes with names like "Paris Green" and "Scheele's Green" that were used to color artificial flowers, fabrics, and wallpaper. The dyes were so popular that by the mid-1800s, England was said to be "bathed" in green with 100 million square feet of arsenic-infused wallpaper. Unfortunately, these products poisoned many of their users by releasing flakes of poisonous paper into the environment or infusing the air with arsenic over time. Once their dangers were understood, they were used as rodenticides. A beautiful dye by-product called London Purple was a fantastic insecticide that also spray-painted plants. Got vermin? Or boring walls? Feeling murderous? Arsenic is your jam.

The death of Napoleon in 1821 has been blamed on many things, including mercury, but high levels of arsenic were found in his hair. Could arsenic have killed him? It might have contributed, but was unlikely the sole cause of death. Samples of wallpaper with those beautiful greens show that they were likely the source. We now know that his nicely decorated prison was probably sickening him.

ARSENIC TODAY

All this talk of poison and toxicity and death! Arsenic as medicine seems like bad judgment in pill form. Worse than, say, flossing with razor wire. But arsenic has actually had a legitimate place in medical history for some time.

Salvarsan, neosalvarsan, and bismarsen are all arsenical compounds that finally brought syphilis to a stop after centuries without a cure. Eventually, penicillin usurped their place. And although older arsenicals were used for the sleeping sickness infection (trypanosomiasis), their toxicity was intolerable. Newer anti-protozoal arsenicals emerged in the twentieth century, but in the 1990s, they were taken off the market once their association with cancer was discovered.

Speaking of cancer, the multipurpose Fowler's Solution was also touted as an anticancer agent. Surprisingly, in this particular realm, it seemed to do some good. In the mid-1800s, it seemed to temporarily stop the signs and symptoms of chronic myeloid leukemia. White arsenic has been used to treat acute promyelocytic leukemia, and is curing many patients today.

Like so many medicines, arsenic has a complex reputation, to say the least. It can be a hero with a homicidal past. (Mary ended up in Sing Sing's electric chair—nicknamed "Old Sparky"—after that fateful third homicide. Murderers can only be so lucky for so long.) It can be a "beautifier" that'll kill you in the process. It can *cause* and *fight* cancer. As Paracelsus once said, "All things are poison and nothing is without poison, only the dosage makes a thing not poison."

Arsenic, it seems, is no exception.

4

GOLD CURE FOR OPIUM HABIT   10.00
GOLD CURE FOR DRUNKENNESS   9.00
GOLD CURE FOR NEURASTHENIA   0.00
REMEDIES SOLD ONLY IN PAIRS

WE BELT THE WORLD.

Gold

Of the Philosopher's Stone, Drunkard's Cures,
Gilded Pills, Heartwarming Drinks,
and Dope for Your Dolls

In 1893, Eugene Lane was found at the entrance to the Brooklyn Bridge late on a Friday night exceptionally drunk. So drunk, in fact, that the police officer described him as "blind and deaf and dumb." He was dragged off to the New York City prison in downtown Manhattan, fondly called The Tombs, and locked up.

The next day, with a searing headache, eyes like a dead fish, and among his "odorous surroundings," Lane was able to explain how he'd ended up in jail. He had just been celebrating a successful alcoholism treatment program with other graduates from the Keeley Institute in White Plains. Or it seemed, not so successful.

Dr. Leslie E. Keeley was a Union Army surgeon who promised a miraculous addiction cure. In 1880, he began treating alcohol and opium addicts in his Dwight, Illinois, sanatorium. Going against the medical status quo, he exclaimed, "Alcoholism is a disease and I can cure it."

And cure it, he *tried*. For years, the trains to Dwight were filled with "sots" desperate for sobriety. After checking in, the patient was immediately given an injection in the arm. A tonic was also prescribed, one teaspoon every two hours. The patients would line up, waiting to get their multiple shots and teaspoons per day with military-like precision.

The formula for the tonic and the injections was proprietary and fiercely protected. In fact, the actual recipe went to the grave with Keeley. But there was one ingredient he proudly and openly advertised—gold.

DRINKABLE GOLD: IMMORTALITY IN A GLASS

Keeley wasn't the first to swear by the curative properties of a gold-flecked tonic. Humans have been trying to consume gold for their health for thousands of years. But here's the rub: More often than not, the body can't do anything with it. When taken orally, pure gold passes right on through, making our stool more sparkly and valuable than it was the day before. For a long time, physicians had no idea what to do with the stubborn

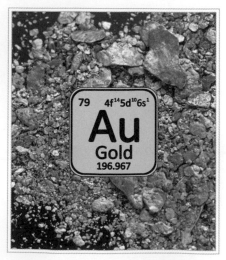

element. It didn't change chemically, didn't mix in solutions, and didn't seem to do anything to anybody. Even some of the most outspoken experts in medicine (Hippocrates, Celsus, and Galen) were quiet on the subject.

So why did we keep trying to consume this beautiful but seemingly useless element?

Immortality, for starters. Of course, luxurious gold is where medical innovation gets greedy. Sure, you reached for antimony when you needed to vomit or for the lancet or leech if you needed to bleed, but sometimes defeating illness wasn't quite enough. When it came to defying death itself, alchemists were repeatedly lured by the glitter of gold.

As far back as 2500 BCE, the Chinese had known that gold was resistant to corrosion and thus associated it with prolonged life. In the third century CE, alchemist Wei Boyang wrote, "Gold is the most valuable thing in the world because it is immortal and never gets rotten. Alchemists eat it, and they enjoy longevity." Trying to consume gold wasn't exactly a new concept. For almost two millennia starting in 202 BCE, the *Bencao gangmu* materia medica included a few gold recommendations such as this one for sores of the mouth and gums: "Cook a gold article with water and gargle with it regularly." Gold-gargle-schläger, anyone?

With the rise of alchemy in medieval times, the quest to create a drinkable form of gold kicked into high gear. The alchemists' main goal? To create the elixir of life, aka the Philosopher's Stone, aka the magical substance that would bestow immortality. (This was before Harry Potter, of course.) Around 1300 CE, an alchemist named Geber finally figured out how to make gold dissolve in a liquid. This *aqua regia* (royal water) was a yellowish-orange lethal mix of nitric and hydrochloric acid that gave off fumes like your average Disney witch's cauldron. Magically, it could dissolve pure gold, and after further processing, produce a salt—gold chloride—that could be drunk when mixed with water. But even though potions of gold chloride were terribly corrosive, it was a breakthrough. For the first time, chemists felt as if they might unlock the life-giving secrets of this glistening metal.

Paracelsus, in particular, rallied around drinkable gold—*aurum potable*—in the sixteenth century. Believing that gold could make the body "indestructible," he might've oversold the element a bit: "Drinkable gold will cure all illnesses, it renews and restores." He claimed it could help with mania, St. Vitus Dance disease, and epilepsy. Also, it "made one's heart happy."

Did it really cure? Hard to say. One thing was for sure, it was definitely toxic. The gold chloride salts could cause kidney damage and something called auric fever,

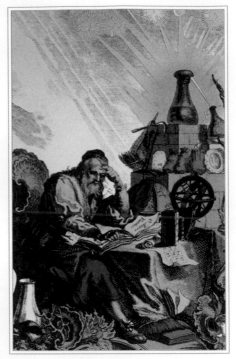

Paracelsus majestically ponders over drinkable gold.

which not only made the sufferer feverish, but also involved profuse salivation and urination.

Maybe people were better off when gold wasn't so drinkable.

GILDED PILLS, EXPLOSIVE CORDIALS, AND OTHER SHINY BAD IDEAS

Oddly enough, physicians—such as seventeenth-century botanist and doctor Nicholas Culpeper—continued to prescribe gold for the same reasons Paracelsus did (sometimes even coating the gold chloride with a layer of gold to make a gilded pill, for extra effect). The drawbacks were a risk patients were willing to take. For those who were suffering from the likes of epilepsy or mental illness, the shimmering promise of gold was still worth a shot.

Unfortunately, many charlatans exploited gold's allure to sell useless medicines. One such salesman was Leonhard Thurneysser zum Thurn. The son of a goldsmith, Thurneysser began his tarnished career in the sixteenth century when he gilded chunks of cheap metal and tried to sell them as pure gold. He eventually decided that practicing medicine was where the money was and started a business creating and selling exorbitantly priced elixirs that claimed to include potable gold with dramatic names like "tincture of gold" and "magistery of the sun," which likely had no soluble gold chloride in them. It was all flash and no medicine. Eventually, a professor in Frankfurt wrote a scathing exposé. Thurneysser lost his business and his riches as well, via a very modern route—a scandalous divorce. Surely, there is a lesson here somewhere.

Although we see gold appear in many seventeenth-century pharmacopeias, it's clear that quacks, rather than real practitioners, were more apt to sell these potions. Doctors, after all, had yet to demonstrate that gold had any beneficial effect on the body. But who cares about a minor thing like empirical findings when you have great marketing? Gold medicine peddlers' favorite promise was that gold possessed "cordiality." Not friendliness, but rather a good and warm effect on the heart (cor = heart, Latin). Because the old alchemists thought that gold represented the sun and the heart was the physiologic equivalent to the sun and warmth, it sort of made sense. Cordials would be made for hundreds of years, bringing warmth (usually via alcohol) to the drinkers, sometimes swimming with flecks of physiologically inert gold particles to make the buyer think they were getting the royal treatment. Certainly, today's imbibers of Goldschläger feel like they're getting a spangled treat!

Even though these salesmen were lying about their products, it might have been for the best. Yes, these tonics and tinctures didn't contain gold, but you probably didn't want the real thing anyway. Besides the fever-inducing salt, alchemists stumbled upon something called fulminating gold, a toxic combination of gold, ammonia, and chlorine. Also touted as a "cordial" heart-warmer, the compound exploded onto the pharmaceutical scene. And we mean that literally: It had a lovely tendency to explode spontaneously. Wonderful for pyromaniacs, not so much for the sick. Sometimes innovation is a bad thing.

By the eighteenth century, gold did the impossible and lost its luster. Physicians started listening to chemists who dismissed the alchemical framework of its medicinal potential. Some like Herman Boerhaave said that it was "of little use in medicine, except for ostentation."

But it would take more than a few critics and explosive cathartics to tarnish this metal. Medicinal gold wasn't finished yet.

Sex, Drugs, and Booze: Gold for STDs and Alcoholism

In the nineteenth century, the desperate search for a cure for syphilis brought gold back onto the medicinal scene. Even though mercury was far more loved when it came to treating the STD, some turned to gold in the form of a less caustic preparation of sodium chloride and gold chloride. Like many medicines treating syphilis at the time, it seemed to work because syphilis symptoms abate on their own. But the power of anecdotal evidence did the job. Gold was back in the form of pills, lozenges, gold salt powders for the gums, and even an injection and tonic that promised to cure an affliction affecting thousands—alcoholism.

Dr. Leslie Keeley was no idiot. In fact, at the time, his idea of treating alcoholism as if it were a disease and not a personal failing was shocking and groundbreaking. But could four injections a day and a slurped tonic really cure thousands of American drunkards? Keeley thought so. He touted a staggering 95 percent cure rate with his gold injections.

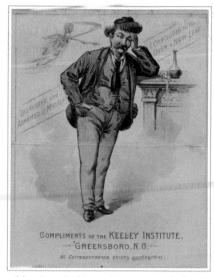

COMPLIMENTS of the KEELEY INSTITUTE,
GREENSBORO, N.G.
All Correspondence strictly confidential

Ad for a branch of the Keeley Institute. The flying skeleton is a nice touch.

First of all, was there even any gold in those injections? It was the most alluring part of his advertising. But Keeley staunchly refused to give up the formula. On a few occasions, he personally provided samples for testing, revealing traces of gold in the injectables.

Secret testing by others without Keeley's permission could not find substantial amounts of gold in either the potion or the injections. What they did find, however, were plenty of interesting ingredients: morphine, cannabis, cocaine, willow bark extracts, and alcohol. Other analyses found strychnine and atropine. At the height of its popularity—it was easily found throughout the United States, either in institutes or by mail order—Keeley's medicine was universally known as "dope" and children would threaten their dolls with "dope" if they didn't get better soon. That would explain why the officers who arrested Eugene Lane said he appeared stupefied and unintelligible by "some o' them drugs they do be takin' up there at Dr. Keeley's."

As for the gold? It seemed to be only gilding on a treatment that might have done more to sedate patients through their tough alcohol withdrawal than actually cure them. Detractors at the time reported their own numbers, claiming that instead of the 95 percent cure rate that Keeley boasted, only about 20 to 50 percent of patients stayed dry initially. Given that there was no compulsory data on long-term follow-up, the final number was likely far lower.

After Keeley's death in 1900, a legal battle ensued between the company and one of his early partners, Fred Hargraves, who claimed that the remedies

LUNACY AND BLUE MEN

Medicinal silver may not have the glitz of gold, but it does have more substance. Used today topically as an antimicrobial, silver was reputed to deter spoilage in ancient times—a reputation that extended to the era of American pioneers, who reportedly dropped silver coins in containers of milk to keep them fresh.

Alchemists connected silver with the mind and the moon (akin to gold's relationship with the sun), giving rise to terms of mental disorders like *lunatic*. The rich who ingested enough silver from their spoons that it changed their skin color were known as "blue-bloods." Like silver lovers of yore, some proponents today consume so much silver to prevent infections that it's turned their skin blue (a condition known as *argyria*). Stan Jones, a Libertarian politician who unsuccessfully ran for Senate and Montana governor twice between 2000 and 2006, had developed a severe case of argyria after drinking large amounts of colloidal silver to

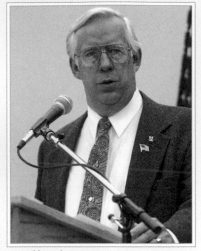

A *true blue Libertarian.*

prepare for Y2K, thinking there would be an antibiotic shortage. Speaking to reporters about his gray-blue skin, he said, "People ask me if it's permanent and if I'm dead. I tell them I'm practicing for Halloween." Or a Smurf parade, perhaps.

---

contained no gold. Early on, he and Keeley had treated one man with a gold formula, and that man had died. Not exactly promising results. But they kept the "gold cure" name. It seemed Keeley was satisfied enough with the idea that "there is a trace of gold in everything, gold in sea water, in mud—everything. There is a trace of gold in it, and that is enough."

Apparently, not all that glitters in advertising is gold. It certainly doesn't cure alcoholics.

Just ask Eugene Lane.

The Modern Gilded Age

Nowadays, people would be surprised to hear that gold actually does have a legitimate place in the medical toolbox. Alas, after all of humanity's efforts in the name of *aurum potable*, those potions were either useless or too toxic. But its other forms have plenty of uses. Colloidal gold—a mixture of microscopic gold and other substances—is used in electron microscopy. We can thank gold alloys for filling our cavities. Gold nanoparticles are being investigated as cancer treatments; they accumulate preferentially in tumor cells, can bind to proteins and drugs, and may enhance the effect of certain therapies.

Gold compounds, either injected or in pill form, have been used in the treatment of rheumatoid arthritis, possibly due to anti-inflammatory properties (the reason isn't completely understood yet). Sometimes these gold compounds have a hefty side effect profile—one of which is *chrysiasis*. That's when gold particles (it takes about eight grams' worth—several years of treatment) accumulate in skin pigment cells and, with exposure to sun, turn the patient a shade of blue-gray. As far as skin goes, physically gilding a human can't really help you, but it can't kill you, either. Remember that James Bond *Goldfinger* scene with the dead, golden woman who died of "skin asphyxiation"? It made for a rather arresting scene, but it was all dazzle and no science.

It's no surprise that the modern usage of medicinal gold is very narrow. All these years, it's been more sparkle than it's worth.

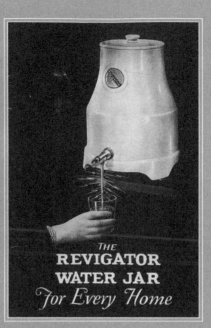

5

THE
**REVIGATOR
WATER JAR**
For Every Home

Radium & Radon

Of Poisoned Playboys, the Curies, Radium Suppositories, and How to Irradiate Your Drinking Water

Late one November evening in 1927, Eben Byers—a forty-seven-year-old industrialist, socialite, and ladies' man—fell from his berth in his private chartered train.

That night he'd been in an exuberant mood, having just watched Yale, his alma mater, defeat Harvard in their annual football match. Buoyed by his team's win, Byers launched the kind of party only a wealthy playboy could host on a private train in the Roaring Twenties (aka the kind of party we all wish we could attend every Friday night).

During the late-night revelry, Byers took a bad fall and injured his arm. When the pain remained with him several days later in the comfort of his mansion, he turned to his handsomely paid physicians. They were stumped. Despite their best efforts, Byers's arm pain would not subside. The injury had a detrimental effect on his serious golf game. (He had won the US Amateur Championship twenty-one years earlier, in 1906.)

Worse for the wealthy playboy, the injury dampened his raging libido.

The notorious womanizer was desperate for solutions. At a loss, one of Byers's physicians suggested he try a new patent medicine called Radithor. Manufactured by Bailey Radium Laboratory in New Jersey, each bottle of Radithor was guaranteed to contain two microcuries of radium, the new kid on the medical block and still blossoming with potential. Radithor was widely advertised as a cure-all for some 150 maladies, including dyspepsia, high blood pressure, and impotence. It also didn't hurt that the doctor, along with every other physician who prescribed Radithor, received a generous 17 percent kickback from the manufacturer.

Byers began taking the medicine. When his arm pain improved, he became convinced that Radithor had increased his vitality. He began drinking three bottles of Radithor a day in December 1927, three times the recommended daily amount. It was a luxury unique to his financial situation because the average person couldn't afford to keep up that kind of dosage. And that was a good thing—by 1931, the industrialist had built up radiation dosage levels equivalent to receiving several thousand X-rays.

Unfortunately for Byers, this level of radiation didn't turn him into a Marvel superhero. It slowly—and gruesomely—killed him.

RADITHOR
REG. U.S. PAT. OFF.
CERTIFIED
Radioactive Water
Contains
Radium and Mesothorium
in Triple Distilled Water

Radithor, with 2 microcuries of radium in triple-distilled water. Byers drank three of these every day.

BEHOLD, THE POWER OF RADIUM!

Famously discovered and isolated by Marie and Pierre Curie—who ultimately gave their health, and in Marie's case, her life, for this scientific breakthrough—radium was embraced by the medical community of the early twentieth century for its striking ability to destroy cancerous cells. Of course, the problem with radium is that it's less like a heat-seeking missile and more like a nuclear bomb. It can affect any cell it encounters, cancerous or not.

Before the dangers of radium were fully understood, however, the element enjoyed a brief life (half-life?) as the celebrity element du jour. In 1902, the Curies first isolated radium chloride from a uranium-rich mineral and ore now called "uranite." (A quick primer: As uranium decomposes, it transforms into other elements. Radium is just a stop on the one-way decomposition train from uranium to lead.) The new element, which Marie called "my beautiful

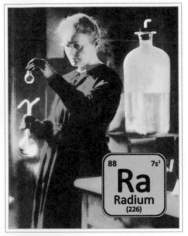

Marie Curie aglow with her "beautiful radium."

radium," glowed with both radioactivity and medical promise. Radium had a half-life of sixteen hundred years and had a radioactivity level of about three thousand times that of uranium. It was enormously rare and enormously intriguing. (And enormously dangerous, but we'll get to that later.)

Less than a year later, while commenting on radium's ability to cause deep flesh burns, Pierre Curie suggested that it might have potential to treat cancer. Initial results were very promising, particularly with skin cancers. The next year, 1904, saw John MacLeod, a physician at Charing Cross Hospital in London, developing radium applicators for treatment of internal cancers as well, which shrank tumors.

It's difficult to overstate the importance of that discovery. After losing the war against cancer for centuries, we finally had an ally. And it even glowed! So it was no surprise that, in addition to treating cancer, physicians in the early twentieth century experimented with using radium for hypertension, diabetes, arthritis, rheumatism, gout, and tuberculosis.

Despite the passage of the Pure Food and Drug Act in 1906, radium remained entirely unregulated because it was classified as a natural element rather than as a drug. And so quacks across the country began exploiting radium's mysterious qualities for their own gain. (Advertisements sprang up in newspapers: "Radiate Youth and Beauty," "Radium is Restoring Health to Thousands," and "Remarkable New Radium Cream Liniment Drives Out Pain from Aching Joints and Muscles *Instantly!*")

The only saving grace was that radium was extremely expensive because of its scarcity. As a result, the vast majority of radioactive products peddled by quacks around the United States did not actually contain any radioactive ingredients at all, a quirk of the supply and demand process that undoubtedly saved hundreds, perhaps thousands, of lives.

Radon, the Revigator, and Other Crocks

The first wave of radioactive products to hit over-the-counter markets were water based. Medical opinion had landed on radon (the gas produced by decomposing radium) as the curative, life-giving property in hot springs that were popular

around the turn of the twentieth century—especially the famous springs in Arkansas (see box, "Radium Spa Hotels," page 55). No one really knew what it was about the hot springs that made them curative, but once the presence of radon was identified, it wasn't much of a leap to assume that radioactivity was responsible. Radon, however, had a serious problem. It can only temporarily remain in water before it either decays or evaporates into the air.

Today, we explicitly try to remove radon from our drinking water (obviously). But in the early twentieth century, a lively trade sprang up in devices built to do the exact opposite. In addition to soaking in radon-laced pools, many people believed drinking radioactive water was generally a good idea, sort of the equivalent of downing a green drink today. One of the most successful devices to add radon to water was the Revigator, invented by R. W. Thomas and patented in 1912. The Revigator was described as a "radioactive water crock," which was essentially true—it was a large jar made of radium-containing uranium ore with an attached spigot. Consumers were instructed to fill the jar every night and "drink freely," averaging between six and seven glasses each day. The Revigator became your very own home radioactive spring, guaranteed to produce a "health-giving drink." And if you had any leftover water at the end of the day? Advertisements encouraged consumers to water their plants!

One of the problems with the Revigator—besides slowly poisoning people with about five times the radium concentration recommended for drinking water—was its lack of portability. Several similar but smaller devices sprang onto the market, including the Thomas Cone, the Zimmer Emanator, and the Radium Emanator, all of which operated on the similar principle that you simply plopped them into water you were about to drink. (These devices, collectively dubbed "emanators," were typically manufactured from carnotite ore, a primary ore of uranium. The uranium would gradually decompose, producing radium and radon gas in turn, which then infused the water to make it radioactive.) At last, you could make radioactive

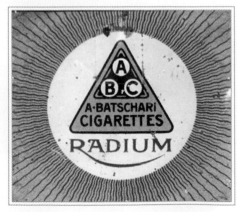

Radium cigarettes, anyone?

water anywhere. Traveling salesmen could rest assured that their drinking water at night in their roadside motel was suitably irradiated.

As the relationship between radon and radium began to be understood more clearly (in terms of radioactive potency, radium is basically radon squared), it wasn't long before manufacturers began to release products allowing consumers to directly consume radium or apply it to their skin. Throughout the 1920s, a variety of radium-based cosmetics were released on the market, including beauty creams, salves, soaps, and toothpaste. Yes, toothpaste. It wasn't enough to have white teeth in the 1920s, those little pearls had to *glow*.

"Ionizing Your Glands" with Jockstraps and Suppositories

Medical controversy reigned over how exactly radioactivity benefited the human body. Some claimed that radium worked by direct application to diseased parts; others thought it stimulated the endocrine system, particularly the adrenal and thyroid glands. For a time, consensus landed on the idea that healthy human functioning relied upon ionizing radiation, that is, X-rays and gamma rays.

Before producing Eben Byers's precious Radithor, William Bailey invented the "Radiendocrinator," a gold-plated harness containing radium that the patient (or victim) could wear around whatever body part was in need of rejuvenation. The Radiendocrinator, you see, produced gamma rays that would "ionize the endocrine glands." The idea was that ionizing (i.e., irradiating) the endocrine system would increase hormone production. Or, as it was better understood by its less enlightened audience, the device worked by "lighting up dark recesses of the body." The Radiendocrinator could even be worn under the scrotum in a special jock strap rigged up to energize uninspired penises.

In 1924, Bailey reached the zenith of his career with a wildly optimistic speech about radium's medicinal potential before the American Chemical

Society. He told them: "We have cornered aberration, disease, old age, and in fact life and death themselves in the endocrines." Bailey believed (or at least claimed to believe, as Bailey's true beliefs are obscured behind his marketing) that aging was caused by the gradual decline of the endocrine glands. By irradiating or "ionizing" them, radium could revitalize them, which in turn would restore some luster to the aged and decrepit. He added:

> I am satisfied from definite clinical experience with the Radiendocrinator that a method of ionization is now available whereby we can definitely, practically without exception, retard the progress of senescence and give a new lease of relatively normal functioning power to those whose sun of life is slowly sinking into the purple shadows of that longest night. . . . The wrinkled face, the drawn skin, the dull eye, the listless gait, the faulty memory, the aching body, the destructive effects of sterility, all spell imperfect endocrine performance.

Bailey wasn't the only one focused on the relationship between radium and glands. Home Products, a company based in Denver, Colorado, had the diabolically brilliant idea of combining animal gland tablets and radium supplements for potent cures to help "weak discouraged men bubble over with joyous vitality."

The men who had the unfortunate experience of taking Vita Radium certainly bubbled over with something, because those radium supplements were suppositories. Radium suppositories. Patients were literally putting radium up their own asses.

The women, however, had it worse. In an effort to combat that eternal feminine problem of "sexual indifference," Home Products produced "Women's Special Suppositories." When inserted vaginally, these radium suppositories were claimed to cure all manner of sexual afflictions and, what's more, reinvigorate their sexual appetites.

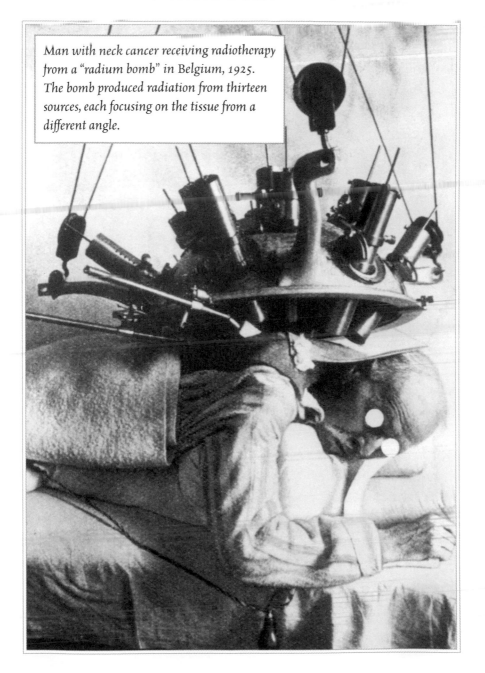

Man with neck cancer receiving radiotherapy from a "radium bomb" in Belgium, 1925. The bomb produced radiation from thirteen sources, each focusing on the tissue from a different angle.

THE GRUESOME DEATH OF AN INDUSTRIALIST

By the end of 1927, Eben Byers, our wealthy industrialist, was routinely drinking several bottles of Radithor each day, convinced it was responsible for the improvement in his health. With all the zeal of a recent convert, Byers began sending cases of Radithor to his friends, colleagues, and female "acquaintances" with his enthusiastic stamp of approval. (One of whom, Mary Hill, preceded him in death, likely from the radiation as well.) He was so completely taken with the patent medicine that he even fed some to his favorite racehorses. For perhaps the only time in history, you could watch a radioactive horse at the tracks in the late 1920s.

Over the next five years, Byers consumed an astonishing fifteen hundred bottles of Radithor. By 1931, his body was literally destroying itself from the inside out. The last eighteen months of his life were straight out of a horror film.

When the once strong and robust ladies' man finally died from the multiple radiation-based cancers raging through his body, on March 31, 1932, he weighed a scant ninety-two pounds. His kidneys had completely failed, leaving his skin sallow and sunken. His brain had abscessed, rendering him nearly mute but entirely lucid. Most of his jaw had been removed by surgeons in failed attempts to stop the spread of cancer. And his skull was riddled with holes from the radiation.

"A more gruesome experience in a more gorgeous setting would be hard to imagine," wrote an observer, commenting on a visit to Byers's Long Island mansion in the final stages of his radiation poisoning. A forensic investigation upon Byers's death revealed that even his own bones were dangerously radioactive. The playboy literally had to be buried in a lead-lined coffin.

Byers's high-profile demise was a watershed moment and led to a full FDA investigation into Radithor and, subsequently, a Federal Trade Commission cease-and-desist order halting its production. Every bottle then available in stores around the country was removed, and government pamphlets were distributed nationally warning about the dangers of consuming the product. By the early 1930s, the formerly lucrative market in radium patent medicines had almost entirely collapsed.

Despite his company receiving the cease-and-desist, Bailey was never actually prosecuted for Byers's death. The scam artist maintained that it was a case of misdiagnosis, citing his own regular consumption of Radithor: "I have drunk more radium water than any man alive, and I have never suffered any ill effects." Bailey slipped off into obscurity, dying in Massachusetts in 1949 at the relatively young age of sixty-four. His cause of death—bladder cancer—was a likely by-product of his own radiation poisoning. Bailey's body, exhumed in 1969, was found to be highly radioactive, so the quack was right about one thing: He practiced what he preached.

Radium Today

Meanwhile, on the legitimate medical front, many of the early radium experimenters (including the Curies) had begun to develop radiation-induced health problems as well. The dangers to the medical field in handling the substance, combined with the dangers to the patients if given imprecise doses, soon overwhelmed its healing potential.

Help came, however, in the form of the Geiger counter in 1928, which allowed scientists to successfully measure radioactivity levels, a crucial safety development as they continued to investigate radium. Radium was applied to tumors by enclosing it in tiny glass tubes, in turn put inside platinum containers, and then plunged into the diseased tissue. The platinum containers block the undesirable alpha and beta rays, while allowing the useful gamma rays through. Similarly, with the introduction of radon sealed in gold tubes (called seeds) in the 1940s, physicians were also able to successfully experiment with radium's decay product. (The gold worked as the platinum did,

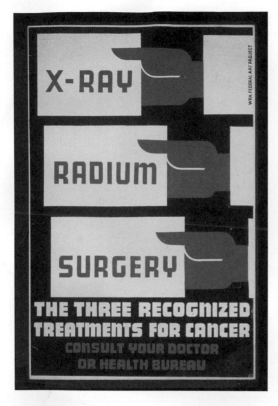

allowing just the gamma rays to escape.) The dangers, however, from leaking gas or contaminated samples, eventually led to the discontinuation of most radium from medicinal use by the 1980s. It still has its place, however—radium[223] is currently a standard therapy for certain stages of prostate cancer. Today, radiation treatment (aka radiotherapy) is most commonly delivered as ionizing radiation beams. In this form, it remains one of the primary treatments for cancer, along with surgery and chemotherapy.

In a curious postscript, in 1989 scientist Roger Macklis investigated the radioactivity of a bottle of Radithor he had purchased at a medical antiques shop and wrote about the surprising results in *Scientific American*: "I assumed that . . . Radithor's residual activity had decayed to insignificance long ago. I was wrong. Tests . . . revealed that almost 70 years after it had been produced, the nearly empty bottle was dangerously radioactive."

The irradiated bones of Eben Byers, slowly decomposing in a lead-lined coffin, underscore that point.

RADIUM SPA HOTELS

Taking a soak in a radioactive spring was a favorite method for absorbing radiation. As it became understood that radon was the gas produced by decomposing radium and that some hot springs emanated that very gas, hotels started popping up nearby so people could get in on the radioactive water action.

At the Radium Spa Hotel in Joachimsthal, Czech Republic, not only could you soak in irradiated water, but you could also inhale radon directly through air tubes connected to a processing tank in the basement. Even the interior air at the hotel was purposefully irradiated.

Another such hotel opened up in Will Rogers's hometown, Claremore, Oklahoma, when a sulfuric spring was discovered and marketed as "radioactive" even though it actually, well, wasn't. But that didn't stop the town and hotel from becoming a major tourist destination in the early twentieth century when radiation was all the rage.

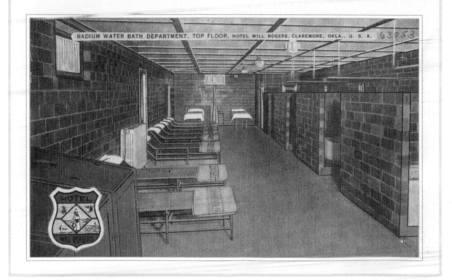

RADIUM WATER BATH DEPARTMENT, TOP FLOOR, HOTEL WILL ROGERS, CLAREMORE, OKLA., U. S. A.

The Women's Health Hall of Shame

Throughout history, the medical care of women has mostly been determined by men. Women have been considered physiologically and psychologically inferior (a sarcastic thanks to Aristotle for asserting that "the woman is a failed man"). Female organs were thought to be the corrupted, inverted version of men's, and women were "leaky vessels" (menstruating, crying, lactating). Menstruating was "polluting."

For millennia, many considered the uterus to be the anatomical and pathological basis of most female ailments. The organ was thought to be extremely high maintenance (even though it self-purged via menses), and it "wandered" hither and thither, causing all sorts of trouble while galloping around the body.

Good God. Get a leash for that womb already. Maybe a shock collar or an electric fence, before it flies off to Bali with some loose testicles.

Meanwhile, we'll take a look at how women's ailments have been treated (poorly) throughout time.

SCENT TREATMENTS

The term *hysteria* (from the Greek word *hystera*, for womb) is actually a more recent term from the 1800s, but the idea of a mischievous, wandering womb goes back to ancient times. Hysteria included symptoms of faintness, insomnia, abdominal discomfort, spasms, loss of interest in sex, increased interest in sex—basically, any problem could be pinned on it. The Ebers Papyrus (1550 BCE) thought that fixing many female problems was a simple matter of making that elusive uterus move back to where it belonged by chasing it about with odors. Uterus "too high" up in the abdomen? Place some stinky feet or other

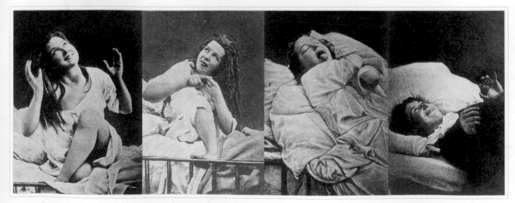

Late-nineteenth-century photos depicting hysteria.

malodorous substances at the nose to drive that organ downward. Or place sweet scents near the vagina to lure it closer. In the nineteenth century, ladies carried around smelling salts (*sal volatile*), with the hope that sniffing them would put that pesky uterus right and—bonus!—prevent a swoon.

HYSTERECTOMIES AND CLITORIDECTOMIES

Surgical removal of the ovaries to treat hysteria began in the nineteenth century. It would be nice to think this was all a clever plan by women wishing to control their own fertility, but the surgery often occurred without the patient's consent. In mid-1880s London, prominent gynecologist Isaac Baker Brown decided that anything that nourished or gratified a woman's sexual appetite was bad, bad, bad. He recommended and performed clitoris removals and even chopped out his sister's ovaries. This clitoridectomy procedure existed into the twentieth century (and is now one of many horrendous procedures termed *female genital mutilation*, still existing in numerous countries). One patient in 1944 had the procedure done and stated, "They tried to keep me from masturbating." She added, "Didn't work."

RED NITRE

For thousands of years, when children could not be produced, the blame has been placed upon women. It didn't help that the biology of human procreation was a mystery for much of this time. For infertility, Hippocrates recommended, "When the cervix is closed too tightly the inner orifice must be opened using a special mixture composed of red nitre, cumin, resin, and honey."

And just what was this red nitre? It might have been potassium nitrate, or saltpeter, which is used for pickling corned beef and making fireworks. Or it could have been soda ash, or natron—what Egyptians used to dry out their mummies. Either way, it was supposed to irritate that cervix into opening wide up. Pickling, fireworks, and mummies. . . . Hmm. Not exactly the most pleasant things you'd want to associate with baby making.

GARLIC CLOVES AND ANISE

According to Hippocrates, other indications of fertility assumed there was an internal freeway communicating between the mouth and the vagina. So, if you rubbed a garlic clove near her nether regions and smelled garlic breath, a woman was obviously fertile. Another fragrant variation included having her drink anise in water; if her belly button itched the next day, she was a baby-making machine raring to go.

ANIMAL REMEDIES FOR CHILDBIRTH

For a successful childbirth, first-century scholar Pliny the Elder recommended putting the right foot of a hyena on the pregnant woman to help with the delivery. (The left foot would cause death. Who knew "lethal hyena left feet" was in the poisoner's armamentarium?) He also advised drinking powdered sow's dung for labor pains. Maybe the smell helped distract the mother-to-be?

Other Pliny pregnancy pairings: Drinking goose semen (okay—how on earth do they ask the male goose to . . . or maybe they just kill the goose and fish out the testicles . . . never mind) or drinking liquids that flowed from a weasel's uterus through its genitals. Yum. How about Pliny's recommendation to use a dog's placenta as a catcher's mitt to pull out the infant being born? Any takers?

BIRD POOP POTION

The *Trotula* is a group of medical texts named after one of its writers, Trota of Salerno, a female physician author who lived in twelfth-century Italy. Before you start celebrating this win for women's rights, read on. She wrote, "If therefore the menses are deficient and a woman's body is emaciated, bleed her from the vein under

the arch of the inside of the foot." To help out a woman giving birth, a potion made from the white stuff found in hawk poop is supposedly useful. Imagine seeing that one written on a prescription pad.

WEASEL NUTS

The *Trotula* also gives contraceptive advice: "Take a male weasel and let its testicles be removed and let it be released alive. Let the woman carry these testicles with her in her bosom and let her tie them in goose skin . . . and she will not conceive." Well. If ever there was a deterrent to sex, it's undressing a woman and finding a pair of weasel nuts shoved betwixt her cleavage. At least it's a good weasel contraceptive. Ah, that poor nutless weasel.

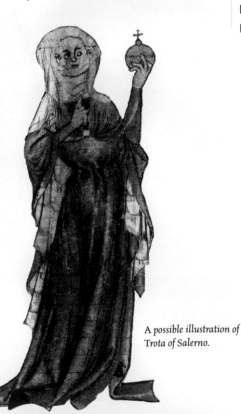

A possible illustration of Trota of Salerno.

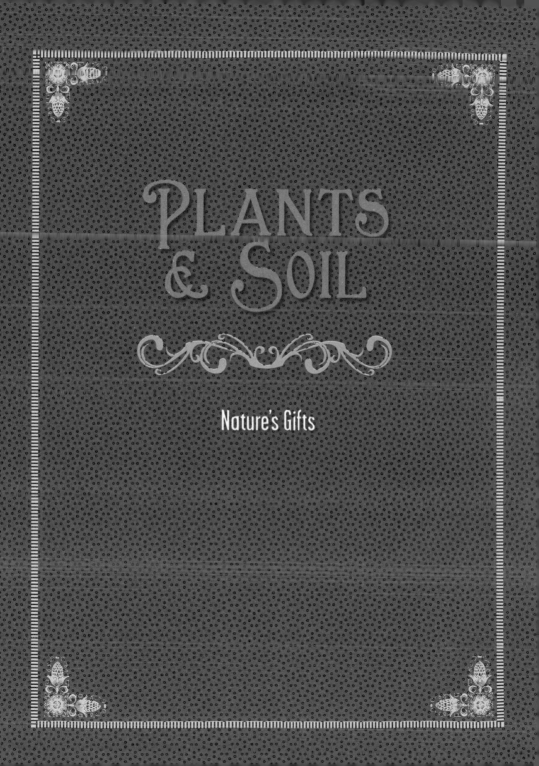

PLANTS & SOIL

Nature's Gifts

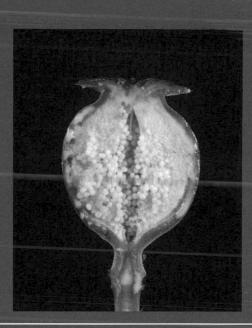

Opiates

Of Poppy-Crowned Gods,
the Stone of Immortality, Heroin the Hero,
and Morphine the Babysitter

Crying infants are not easy on the ears. Especially if you're an overworked baby-minder a century or so ago caring for ten children, whose mothers were working in the local factory. Or you're an older child with little siblings to watch. Or you're an exhausted mother who can't deal with another sleepless night, perhaps with another baby on the way. Sure, those cries are a message that they might be hungry or covered in poop. Maybe it's colic or teething pain. But for crying out loud, *the noise*. One pair of hands can only do so much.

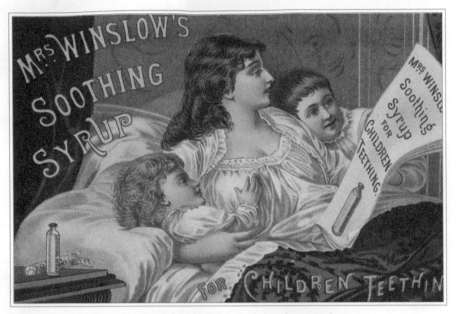

Ah, a mother's bliss of realizing she can finally knock out her kids and get some sleep.

So you might reach for Mrs. Winslow's Soothing Syrup, Godfrey's Cordial, Jayne's Carminative Balsam, or Daffy's Elixir, all containing morphine or opium and all putting that baby right to sleep . . . or killing it.

You might think this is horrible, but drugging noisy infants was standard practice for several millennia. The Ebers Papyrus (1550 BCE) describes using poppy plants mixed with wasp droppings to soothe a crying child. Seventh-century physician and philosopher Avicenna recommended a poppy, fennel, and anise seed potion. From the 1400s until this past century, textbooks recommended varying concoctions with opium and morphine for both sleeplessness and teething. If the baby didn't want to be weaned? Founding father Alexander Hamilton had something to say about it. He recommended "a little weak white-wine whey, diluted brandy punch, or even a tea-spoonful or two of syrup of poppy . . . to prevent restlessness and fits of crying, till the breast is forgotten."

The problem was everywhere. In Edinburgh in the late 1800s, Charles Routh noted that wet nurses were prone to drugging their charges, or themselves. "Either the nurse herself is a dram drinker or opium eater and so far affects the milk by the pernicious habit . . . or, secondly, she drugs the child." The babies slept, sure, but that also meant they didn't eat often, and any illnesses they did have were doped into silence.

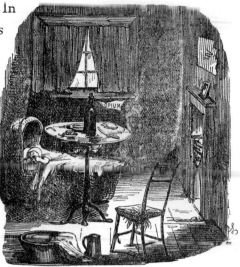

Opium, the poor child's nurse.

THE SWEET LULL(ABY) OF OPIUM

So these babysitters weren't winning any childcare awards. Still, they were taking part in the ancient tradition of utilizing the many properties of opium. Within half an hour of consuming it, you feel euphoric and drowsy, while even your most excruciating pain is numbed away. Sounds wonderful, right? Just wait for the side effects: itchy skin, constipation, nausea, and dangerously slow breathing. Oh, also crippling addiction. And death.

The opium poppy, *Papaver somniferum* (Greek for "poppy" and Latin for "sleep inducing"), has been known to man for more than five thousand years. The flower is a paperish wisp of white, red, pink, or purple, with petals that hardly last two days before withering away on the wind. But don't be fooled by its delicacy: The poppy's power isn't in its flowering beauty, but in the stiff narcotic-laden pod it leaves behind. In 3400 BCE, the Sumerians called it *Hul Gil*, or the "joy plant." Two thousand years later, opium use had

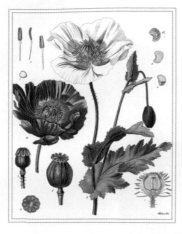

Opium poppy and pods, including cross-section showing laticifer full of opiates.

spread through North Africa, Europe, and the Middle East. Mixed with licorice or balsam, it was said to cure everything. In ancient Egypt, the goddess Isis was rumored to have given opium to the god Ra for his headaches. Because even gods get headaches, right?

In ancient Greece, the divinities were often portrayed with poppies in hand or wreathed as crowns. Opium was associated with a host of gods who offered various forms of sweet relief: Nyx (night), Hypnos (sleep), Thanatos (death), and Morpheus (dreams).

In the fourth century BCE, Hippocrates held an appropriate regard for its dangers and recommended it be used sparingly to sleep, to stop bleeding or pain, and for women's diseases. Homer wrote of a drug that was likely based on opium, called *nepenthe*, which was given to Telemachus by Helen to induce forgetfulness. Hemlock and opium were used in a lethal combination to kill the condemned. Opium was rather useful. But it was misused, all too often.

Galen, in the second century CE, loved opium as a medicinal a little too much. He thought it would cure vertigo, deafness, epilepsy, strokes, bad vision, kidney stones, leprosy, and oh, pretty much everything. After all, it certainly made people feel better. In the seventh century, Avicenna wrote a thesis on opium expounding its benefits. His writings in his *Canon of Medicine* made perfect sense—it can help with painful gout, slow diarrhea, and put insomniacs to sleep. In the latter sense, opium is one of the oldest known hypnotics in the world. He even thought it helped those with out-of-control libidos: "Patients with disturbingly high libido can use opioids topically." Uh, okay.

Avicenna warned his readers about the symptoms of opium toxicity he had observed—difficulty breathing, itching, and unconsciousness. It's easy to imagine, without regulation of dosing or production, that overdoses weren't uncommon, hence Avicenna's words of caution. But in an ironic turn, he succumbed to what was likely the first documented opium overdose in history. Apparently, he was suffering from colic and his servant overdosed his medicine in an effort to steal from him. Oh, he was also having a little too much sex at the time (so much for the lower-libido theory). He died shortly thereafter. (Note to self: Colic plus excessive sex and opium can kill you. Perhaps there are worse ways to die.)

Opium Gets an Upgrade: Laudanum

You can thank Paracelsus for opium's explosion in fifteenth-century Europe. The celebrity physician called opium the stone of immortality and is credited with inventing laudanum, which he humbly declared "superior to all other heroic remedies." One of his contemporaries, Johannes Oporinus, said, "He had pills which he called laudanum which looked like pieces of mouse shit. . . . He boasted he could, with these pills, wake up the dead."

Paracelsus's mouse-poop laudanum (from the Latin, *laudare*: "to praise") was supposedly concocted of 25 percent opium, plus mummy (you read that correctly: see Cannibalism & Corpse Medicine, page 221), bezoar stone taken from a cow's digestive tract, henbane (a sedative and hallucinogenic plant), amber, crushed coral and pearls, musk, oils, the bone from the heart of a stag (what?), and unicorn horn (more likely, rhinoceros or narwhal). Some of his recipes included frog spawn; others called for orange juice, cinnamon, cloves, ambergris, and saffron. Basically, it was mostly

Paracelsus, inventor of laudanum.

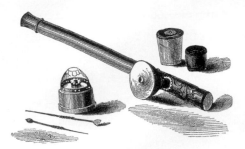

An opium smoker's tools.

opium mixed with a lot of expensive crap that smelled (mostly) awesome. Not a huge improvement on the status quo. Could it wake the dead? Er, no.

In the 1600s, Thomas Sydenham popularized his own take on laudanum, without the frills and furbelows of Paracelsus's version but with one key addition: lots of alcohol. He included tasty additions of cinnamon and cloves, too. It was touted as a treatment for the plague. Sadly, laudanum didn't *cure* the plague. But it probably made victims feel a lot better while the disease mercilessly killed them. Not that Sydenham would know—he fled London to avoid the plague like . . . uh, the plague.

Meanwhile, opium became a huge commodity across the world. Two opium wars were fought in the nineteenth century. The issues of Chinese sovereignty, addiction, and trade deals swirled in a power play that resulted in the loss of Hong Kong to the United Kingdom for more than 150 years. Opium dens where one could smoke solid opium opened internationally, often supplied through the Chinese opium trade.

But it was laudanum, the liquid version, that took a larger toll in the West. Even though they weren't as potent as straight opium, these derivative medicines packed a punch and tasted better, too. The addition of alcohol only intensified the euphoric and mind-altering effects. The products were touted by most physicians and obtainable without a prescription, used in the comfort of the home—no

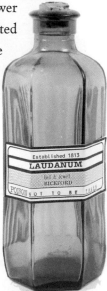

Laudanum— with the warning "not to be taken," which is all sorts of confusing.

opium den required. It was much easier to dose up or down, or up, up, up, as could often be the case.

Inevitably, such an easily affordable medicine brought the dark shadow of addiction along for the ride. It was a soporific that temporarily banished all that was difficult in every class of society. In the 1821 book *Confessions of an English Opium-Eater*, author Thomas De Quincey waxed poetic on his addiction to laudanum. "Here was a panacea . . . for all human woes . . . happiness may now be bought for a penny." And then there was the bad: "I seemed every night to descend . . . into chasms and sunless abysses . . . amounting at last to utter darkness, as of some suicidal despondency."

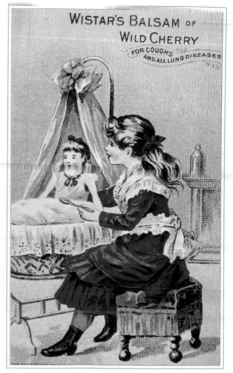

Ad for balsam containing cherry bark, alcohol, and opiates (c. 1840). For "all lung diseases" and playtime, apparently.

Addiction was no joke, and yet druggists sold gallons of laudanum, opium elixirs, and narcotic nostrums. Take Dover's Powder, an eighteenth-century remedy containing opium, ipecac, licorice, saltpeter (potassium nitrate, great for explosives and pickling pork), and vitriolic tartar (potassium sulfate, a fertilizer). While treating colds and fevers, Dover's Powder could put people to sleep . . . permanently. Of the effective dose—seventy grains—creator Thomas Dover said, "Some apothecaries have desired their patients to make their wills before they venture upon so large a dose."

Well, sign us up!

MORPHINE: DREAM OR NIGHTMARE?

Friedrich Wilhelm Adam Sertürner was a mere twenty-one years old when he successfully extracted morphine from the gums and waxes inside the poppy pod. It was 1806. He wasn't even trained in chemistry, only apprenticed to a pharmacist since he was sixteen. His equipment was crude, but he persevered. He called his newly discovered compound *principium somniferum* for the sleep-making principle within opium. And then he named it after the Greek god of dreams—Morpheus.

Say hi to morphine. Of course, Sertürner had to test it. Previously, with his less pure extracts, he'd try them on random dogs and a mouse that had wandered into his lab. This time, he treated himself (ethicists, look away) as well as some teenage boys (IRBs, also look away). He reported, "The outcome with the three young men was decidedly rapid and extreme. It presented as . . . exhaustion, and severe narcosis that came close to fainting. . . . I fell into a dream-like state." Fearful of their degree of intoxication, he had them all drink vinegar to vomit it all up. Some kept vomiting and the intoxicated sensation lasted for days.

Still, he made his point. The extract was indeed what made opium so alluring (and nauseating). And because society is always ready for something stronger and purer, morphine was soon widely available. Sir William Osler, one of the founding fathers of modern medicine, called morphine "God's own medicine." There we go again with gods and their headaches. Though more likely, he meant a creation for man that was unlike any other.

In the nineteenth century, bleeding, purging, leeching, and enemas were still all the rage, but in morphine doctors found something much gentler. Together with opium, it would occupy materia medica texts forever after, recommended for obvious ailments like pain and diarrhea. (Cholera and dysentery killed far fewer people, thanks to opium.) But the medicines were also thrown at anything that ailed people. Snake bites, rabies, tetanus, ulcers, diabetes, poisoning, and depression and other mental illnesses were "cured." Doctors and their patients had found a very comfortable medicine in morphine.

Huge amounts of opium and morphine were used during the Civil War, where they helped with dysentery and terrible battlefield wounds, but also created addicts (so many, that opiate addiction was dubbed soldier's disease or army disease at the time). While still mounted on his horse, Union surgeon Major Nathan Mayer would pour morphine doses into his gloved hand and let soldiers lick it off.

And in the 1850s, just when we thought opium had reached its most potent, accessible form, Alexander Wood invented the modern hypodermic syringe. Injected morphine was stronger and required a far smaller dose. As a result, use became even more widespread, especially in the middle and upper classes because morphine, syringes, and needle kits were expensive.

By the 1880s, Wood's invention brought on new creations: *morphinomania* and *morphinism*, terms for morphine addiction. The syringe was a miracle for medicine, but unfortunately a vehicle for a dark disease.

Heroin, the Hero?

If opium was a euphoric, painkilling gift to humanity, then surely morphine was even better—a godsend. But opium and morphine were creating addicts. So naturally, humankind wasn't satisfied. Our instinct to tinker with nature and look for the next best/horrific thing couldn't be suppressed. Somewhere between the invention of the rocket (thirteenth century) and email (1971), we invented the monster that is heroin.

In 1874 London, a pharmacist named Charles Romley Alder Wright was searching to create a version of morphine without the addictive qualities. His new opiate, diacetylmorphine, was shockingly potent, but it took another decade before a German chemist working for Bayer Laboratories, Heinrich

Dreser, would look to this drug as the winning racehorse that would be Bayer's money-maker.

Another Bayer chemist, Felix Hoffmann, had just "reinvented" aspirin. But Dreser didn't think aspirin would be profitable. It would be "enfeebling" to the heart, he thought. (Everyone out there with coronary artery disease taking aspirin—please ignore that.) So he had Hoffmann whip up some diacetylmorphine instead, knowing it had already been synthesized. He tested it on rabbits and frogs, and then thoughtfully tried it on employees at Bayer. They loved it. Some said it made them feel mighty, or *heroisch* ("heroic," German).

They called it *heroin*. Surely, heroin would be nonaddictive. Surely, this was the new pain reliever everyone was looking for to replace opium. (Never mind that aspirin was, and still is, a great pain reliever.) They even thought it had fewer side effects. And it was potent; almost eight times more so than morphine, which means that smaller amounts could be used. And the kicker?

Bayer touted heroin as a *cure* for morphine addiction.

By 1899, the company was synthesizing a ton of heroin annually, in the form of pills, powders, elixirs, and sweetened lozenges that were sold internationally. Bayer claimed it could treat tuberculosis, asthma, colds, and coughs from all causes. Ads featured effervescent claims: "Heroin clears the complexion, gives buoyance to the mind, regulates the stomach and the bowels, and is, in fact, a perfect guardian of health." Many doctors drank the veritable Kool-aid about heroin being non-addictive. The *Boston Medical Journal* wrote in 1900, "It possesses many advantages over morphine. . . . It is not a hypnotic," and luckily, there was "an absence of danger of acquiring

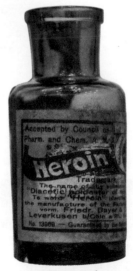

Bayer, a company many don't realize marketed heroin.

the habit." But reality reared its ugly head, and early in the twentieth century, more and more medical journals reported on heroin's dark, addictive side.

OPIATES' DOWNFALL AND PERSISTENCE

Abuse of opium continued into the twentieth century, until the international community decided to finally put their foot down. In 1912, the Hague International Opium Convention promised to usher in an era of drug control. Bayer stopped production of heroin in 1913. The United States followed with its own Harrison Narcotics Act in 1914, which regulated the import, sale, and distribution of opiate and coca products.

An era of conspicuous and socially acceptable opiate consumption was over. Mrs. Winslow's Soothing Syrup would no longer be as easy to procure as a quart of milk. In 1924, the United States banned heroin once and for all.

But it didn't matter. A generation was already hooked, and more would follow. The safeguards of laws and prescribing restrictions still don't stop opioid deaths. In 2015, thirty-three thousand people died in the United States from opioid use, and half of those were taking prescription painkillers.

Medications to reverse opioid overdoses, like Narcan, are widely available outside of emergency departments with and without a prescription. But it's only a temporary fix. Society continues to battle illegal drugs as well as the treacherous balance between pain control and deadly side effects. As long as vast poppy fields still exist, and modern medicine can't produce a safer class of medicines to kill pain, the battle will continue.

So the next time you see Bayer aspirin on the shelves of your supermarket, you'll know how it was overshadowed in its infancy by heroin, the so-called hero that ended up being the villain of the addiction world.

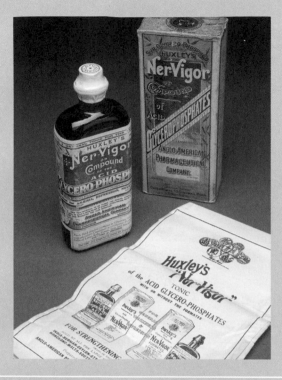

7

Strychnine

Of Poisoned Marathoners, Deadly Trees, Sexual Stimulants, Nefarious Brewers, and Indian Weightlifters

On a hot and humid Missouri day in 1904, a hodgepodge of runners lined up at the start of the Olympic marathon. Their ranks included a debt-ridden Cuban postmaster who had hitchhiked to the event, two African tribesmen who just happened to be in town as part of a Boer War exhibition, and the American distance runner Thomas Hicks.

The race started and ended in the St. Louis stadium, but was otherwise run entirely on Missouri country roads. The heat was in the 90s. With numerous hills and poor roads made worse by the clouds of dust stirred up from passing motorists, the 1904 marathon course was probably the toughest in Olympic history.

As for aid stations? There was a well somewhere around mile eleven.

A stone well. Like, with a bucket.

So Hicks, our American boy, was suffering badly at mile fourteen when his trainers decided to give him a little boost. Performance-enhancing drugs, far from being banned, were still widely used in athletic competitions at the time. Hicks's trainers mixed 1904's equivalent of an energy drink: a 1 milligram dose of strychnine (yes, strychnine) with egg whites to subdue its extreme bitterness. He drank it and carried on running.

Even when Hicks had a generous mile-long lead on his closest competitor, he was slowing down with each grueling hill. Then there was the mounting dehydration. His trainers had denied him drinking water throughout the race, generously offering instead to wash out his mouth with "warm distilled water." So when another dose of strychnine was in order for their struggling runner, Hicks's trainers obviously couldn't mix it with water. Their solution? A strychnine and brandy cocktail.

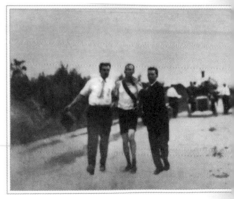

The thrilling conclusion of the 1904 Olympic marathon!

Hicks, in some miracle of human endurance, managed to push on. In the last two miles, a race official wrote that he was "running mechanically, like a well-oiled piece of machinery. His eyes were dull, lusterless; the ashen color of his face and skin had deepened; his arms appeared as weights well tied down; he could scarcely lift his legs, while his knees were almost stiff."

Yeah, that's because the runner was almost dead. Hicks was, by this point, bordering on a toxic level of strychnine poisoning. Combined with the August heat, crippling dehydration, and the sheer physical exertion of running a marathon at an Olympic level, Hicks was quite literally dying. His trainers—shockingly—debated giving him a third dose of strychnine, a move which would almost certainly have killed him.

In the final stretch, he required the physical support of his trainers to keep him in an upright position. A surviving photo of Hicks at that moment shows a strained, rigid expression on his face. That would be the strychnine intoxication, which produces sustained spasms of the facial muscles. Limping, hallucinating, and eight pounds lighter than when he started, Hicks was declared the winner of the 1904 marathon.

STRYCHNINE ENERGY DRINKS

Although they seem absurd today, Hicks's trainers believed, along with the wider medical community of the early twentieth century, that strychnine could increase energy. And they weren't entirely wrong. In small doses, strychnine operates as a short-term stimulant, providing a jolt to the nervous system similar to caffeine. Unlike caffeine, however, it doesn't take much strychnine to kill you. Five milligrams, to be exact.

Because of that strength, strychnine has also been used since the medieval era as a particularly effective—and particularly brutal—method of poisoning rats, cats, dogs, and other unwanted creatures. By preventing the effective operation of glycine—the chemical that sends nerve signals to the muscles—a high dose of strychnine causes severe, painful muscle spasms. Left unchecked, these spasms build in frequency and strength, killing the victim within a few hours through either asphyxiation or sheer exhaustion from the brutal convulsions.

In short, just the thing for a little Olympic marathon pick-me-up.

Or a potent energy drink for a student cramming for an exam.

Strychnine, briefly functioning as a Victorian version of Adderall, made some waves among ambitious medical students of the late nineteenth century trying to defeat the need for sleep. Leonard Sandall, however, went a little too far with his strychnine dosage in 1896. Although he lived to tell the tale, it was not a pleasant experience:

> Three years ago I was reading for an examination, and feeling "run down." I took 10 minims [about 0.02 fluid ounces] of strychnia solution (B.P.) with the same quantity of dilute phosphoric acid well diluted twice a day. On the second day of taking it, toward the evening, I felt a tightness in the "facial muscles" and a peculiar metallic taste in the mouth. There was great uneasiness and restlessness, and I felt a desire to walk about and do something rather than sit still and read. I lay on the bed and the calf muscles began to stiffen and jerk. My toes drew up under my feet, and as I moved or turned my head flashes of light kept darting across my eyes. I then knew something serious was developing . . . My whole body was in a cold sweat, with anginous attacks in the precordial region, and a feeling of "going off." . . . A little time after I lost consciousness and fell into a "profound sleep," awaking in the morning with no unpleasant symptoms, no headache, &c., but a desire "to be on the move" and a slight feeling of stiffness in the jaw. These worked off during the day.

And that, in a nutshell, is what the early stages of strychnine poisoning feel like. Surviving reports of these experiences are quite scarce in the historical record because, well, you have to survive to write a report. Sandall was lucky. Many people weren't.

THE PLANT BEHIND THE POISON

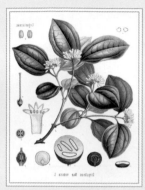

The strychnine alkaloid occurs naturally in the seeds of the strychnine tree (*Strychnos nux-vomica*), a deciduous tree native to India and Southeast Asia. The medium-sized tree grows to forty feet in height and looks rather innocently like an overgrown pear tree. Its flowers have a distinctly unpleasant odor and are replaced by spherical fruits, each of which contains five seeds enveloped by white pulp.

Every single part of the strychnine tree is poisonous. Even parasitic plants that attach themselves to the tree absorb significant quantities of poison. In 1840, an English sailor was recovering from gonorrhea in a Calcutta hospital. Bored and morally bankrupt, the sailor took to beating the hospital's servants during his ample downtime.

Everyone's favorite patient was soon offered a new medicine for his ailment: the powdered leaf of kuchila molung, a parasitic plant that attaches itself to the strychnine tree.

Four hours later, the sailor was dead. Hospital staff wrote off the incident as an "unfortunate mistake."

STRYCHNINE ENEMAS AND OTHER SHOCKS TO THE SYSTEM

Although strychnine tree seeds had been trickling into Europe and used as an animal poison since the medieval period, it wasn't until 1811 that their human medical potential was seriously investigated by Dr. Pierre Fouquier in Paris. The plant had been largely ignored by French doctors until Fouquier theorized that strychnine's almost electric jolt of energy might shock the limbs of paralytic patients into normal operation again.

Armed with an alcoholic extract of strychnine, Fouquier forced himself upon sixteen paralyzed patients at the Hôpital de la Charité. He began his experiments with a thirty-four-year-old male upholsterer, who was confined to his bed under a strange and spreading paralysis that began in his extremities and worked its way up to his pelvis. Fouquier dosed the upholsterer with the extract, first to little effect, but soon, with increased quantities, the patient began to suffer convulsions that appeared to have "shocked" his system into normal functioning. After three months, during which he consumed 314 grains of strychnine, the upholsterer sat up in bed and walked out of the hospital, his paralysis gone. (Probably not a moment too soon.)

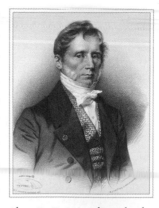

Above: Dr. Fouquier taking a break from poisoning patients. Below: Strychnine correctly labeled as poison!

Fouquier's other experiments were less successful. Consider the unfortunate M. Vanhove, who was singled out for strychnine enemas (let that sink in for a moment). Vanhove, remarkably, was reported as making some progress with his paralysis, when he was accidentally given strychnine pills in addition to the enema. Although he—shockingly—didn't die from the horrific convulsions that soon followed, Vanhove was abruptly written out of Fouquier's account after his health stopped improving.

Fouquier's disturbing experiments encouraged other French scientists to investigate further, and in 1818 the strychnine alkaloid was first isolated from the seeds. French doctors launched a vigorous series of experiments to investigate the efficacy of pure strychnine as a medicine. It didn't turn out so well. The usual dose of strychnine was between 1 and 3 milligrams; however,

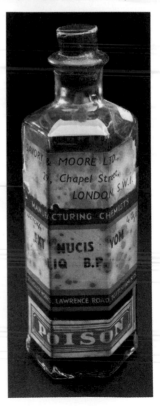

scientists quickly realized that as little as 5 milligrams can produce a fatal poisoning. It was easy to go too far. And many doctors did.

The extraordinary risks of taking strychnine would soon overwhelm its potential as a medicine. While strychnine was falling out of favor in the hospital, however, it was rising in popularity in the pharmacy and on the streets.

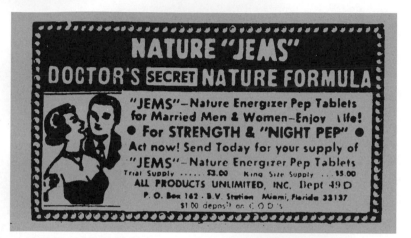

Their euphemism game is strong: Get some "night pep" with strychnine energy pills!

GETTING IT UP WITH STRYCHNINE

After the strychnine alkaloid was extracted, it wasn't long before French scientists started experiments on its sexual applications. The idea was to benefit from the sensory boost kicked in by a small dose. This wasn't an entirely new concept: Rumors of the plant's sexual properties had followed its import into Western markets from India and Southeast Asia in the Victorian era. "I have heard, of some of the more debauched among the Rajpoots, using the nux vomica as a stimulus," wrote an observer in India in the 1830s.

Doctors Trosseau and Pidioux recorded the case of a twenty-five-year-old man who had for eighteen months been able to engage in only "fraternal communication" with his wife. While under the influence of strychnine, the man was able to rise to the occasion, an ability he lost again after he stopped taking the drug. In the pre-Viagra world, you could at least rely on strychnine.

In the 1960s, the Miami-based company All Products Unlimited stumbled upon the old Victorian reputation of strychnine as a sexual stimulant. Hoping to take advantage of the budding sexual revolution, they released a supposed aphrodisiac called Jems in 1966. Awkwardly advertised as "Nature Energizer Pep Tablets for Married Men & Women," Jems included small doses of strychnine in each pill.

The company was soon hauled into court on charges of mail fraud, not for including strychnine in their ingredients list, mind you, but for making baseless claims about the sexual benefits of taking Jems. The company didn't bother to fight the charges and was promptly indicted.

STRYCHNINE IN THE DICTATOR'S MEDICINE CABINET

When strychnine went mainstream, plenty of shysters swept in to profit from this energizing new drug. Fellows & Company, a father and son team that began in Canada and later emigrated to London, produced several dubious household remedies such as Worm Lozenges, Dyspepsia Bitters, and the marvelously vague Golden Ointment. The company did indeed strike gold, however, with the development of Fellows' Compound Syrup of Hypophosphites, an enormously popular patent medicine in the early twentieth century that included strychnine in its contents. Boosted by a personal testimonial from James Fellows himself, who claimed to have been a victim of "secondary stage pulmonary consumption" (i.e., tuberculosis) before his use of the syrup completely cured him, the product was an instant success.

Fellows' Syrup was advertised to be effective "in the treatment of anemia, neurasthenia, bronchitis, influenza, pulmonary tuberculosis and wasting diseases of childhood, and during convalescence from exhausting disease."

BITTER BREWS: SCANDALS OF STRYCHNINE-LACED BEER

In 1851, rumors began circulating that a major British beer producer, Allsopp's Ales, was adulterating their IPAs with strychnine to increase the bitterness. India Pale Ales, as all beer-hounds know, are very hoppy, very bitter ales. Allsopp's was accused of supplementing hops in their brews with strychnine, a cheaper, more poisony alternative.

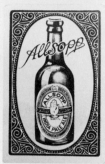

The rumors were rampant enough that Henry Allsopp himself commissioned an independent report by two prominent British chemists to prove that Allsopp ales did not in fact contain any strychnine, a statement that challenges the age-old mantra "There's no such thing as bad press."

In what must have been a surprise to someone somewhere, the British chemists found Allsopp's Ales to be strychnine-free. So Allsopp was off the hook for any pending mass-poisoning charges. But the basis for that rumor had some truth to it. While Allsopp's Ales did not lace their beer with strychnine, pub owners throughout Britain did. Frequently. In the nineteenth century, a pub owner sold beer to his customers at the same cost he paid the brewer. So how could he make a profit? Well, he could water the beer down, sure, but he wouldn't keep his customers very long. But what if there was a way to water the beer down without it tasting watered down?

Enter strychnine.

This magical powder, dissolvable in water, adds the bitterness associated with hops and provides an intoxicating impact similar to unadulterated beer. In other words, just the thing for the greedy pub owner anxious to make a profit. More than a few British alcoholics died from a different type of intoxication in the nineteenth century.

By creating a marketing plan heavily reliant upon the strength of "testimonials," the Fellows company made a tidy profit from their over-the-counter strychnine formula, which sold for seven shillings per 15-ounce bottle. The price was rather exorbitant by the standards of the day, but the crimson gelatin seal on the bottle (pause for "oohs" and "ahs") made it all worth it.

Although not quite as popular, a competing tonic called Easton's Syrup contained about twice the amount of strychnine as Fellows'. At 6 fluid ounces per pint in 1911, it took only a quarter of a pint to produce a fatal dose.

Another strychnine tonic called Metatone was launched in 1930 and included $^1/_{25}$ grain strychnine per ounce. Still easily procurable today in the United Kingdom, Metatone is advertised as a tonic to restore health and vitality after an illness. Strychnine, however, is noticeably absent from its ingredients list, having been quietly removed in 1970.

Strychnine also crept its way into a German drug for digestion problems called Dr. Koester's Antigas Tablets. In the early 1940s, Dr. Theodor Morell began prescribing these tablets to one of his patients who suffered from constipation and flatulence from a vegetarian diet. The doctor recommended his patient take between eight and sixteen tablets per day, which he did, faithfully, for nine years, until he took his own life in a bunker beneath Berlin at the conclusion of World War II.

Yes, Adolf Hitler was consuming near-lethal doses of strychnine during his reign of terror. Over time, the strychnine powder would have accumulated in larger and larger quantities in his intestines and, in turn, possibly led to the increasingly erratic behavior Hitler demonstrated as he neared the end of his life.

STRYCHNINE'S DOWNFALL

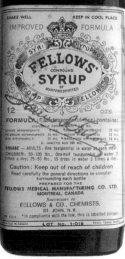

By the early 1970s, strychnine was finally creeping out of fashion, as arguments in the *British Medical Journal* advocated for its complete removal from any use in human medicine.

Today, strychnine is shunned in the West, but we still test for it in the urine of athletes. A century after Hicks's race, strychnine doping surfaced again in 2001 when an Indian weightlifter was banned from competition for six months after strychnine was found in her urine. That athlete, Kunjarani Devi, also had to return a gold medal she had won at an Asian weightlifting competition. Devi made the dubious claim that she had simply drunk too much coffee. She argued, without scientific basis, that strychnine occurs in small quantities in coffee. More likely Devi had taken a large dose of nux vomica, still a widely available homeopathic remedy in India.

Devi was not totally off-base, though. Although the strychnine alkaloid is not actually found in coffee, caffeine is very present in our favorite morning beverage. And caffeine and strychnine are remarkably similar molecules. Both operate as a glycine inhibitor in the human body. Strychnine is just stronger. A lot stronger.

So if you ever want to experience a feeling mildly akin to strychnine poisoning, try downing a few pints of strong coffee. As your heart races, your senses quicken, and your muscles twitch, you can enjoy that same stimulative kick chased by French medical students in the nineteenth century and Olympic marathoners in the twentieth . . . without the unfortunate side effects of horrific convulsions and agonizing death.

But then again, you might get a heart arrhythmia and end up in the ER, so it may be better to just stick to a thought experiment.

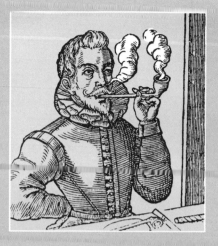

8

Tobacco

Of Cigarette Prescriptions, Creamy Snuff, and Blowing Smoke Up Your Ass

"More doctors smoke Camels than any other cigarette!"

"20,679 physicians say Luckies are less irritating!"

"Give your throat a vacation, smoke a fresh cigarette!"

Such were the effusive claims for the health benefits of cigarette smoking, found in colorful advertisements in magazines around the country in the early to mid-twentieth century. Was it any wonder that more than 50 percent of the adult male population smoked in 1955? Physicians themselves were avid smokers; around the same time, 30 percent of doctors reported smoking at least a pack of cigarettes a day.

Two generations later and, in the United States anyway, smoking levels are now at historic lows. It's a seismic shift in sixty years for a highly addictive substance that people were convinced was a health aid for the previous five centuries.

But don't get us wrong: Tobacco is still the deadliest plant known to mankind, directly responsible for more than 6 million deaths each year worldwide. Although widely recognized today as a killer, tobacco also has a long history as a medicinal herb and was embraced in both the Old and New Worlds for its healing properties well into the twentieth century.

Joyful News out of the New Found World

Native to the Americas, the sixty species of *Nicotiana* have been cultivated for thousands of years. By the time Spanish explorers arrived in the fifteenth century, tobacco was in widespread use across both North and South America as a ritual aid, a recreational drug, and a medicinal herb.

Members of Columbus's crew observed the indigenous Taíno people of present-day Cuba and Haiti burning tobacco leaves in torches to ward off diseases and disinfect homes and ritual places. The crew also reportedly saw the Taíno snuff large quantities of dried tobacco, a process that resulted in a quick loss of consciousness and was possibly employed by local physicians as a way to knock someone out before conducting trepanning surgery. (While there remains some debate about the origin of the word *tobacco*, the Taíno word for either the tobacco leaves themselves or for the pipe used to smoke them is a strong contender.)

Later explorers continued to observe widespread medicinal use of tobacco across the New World. In Mexico, it was employed as an antidiarrheal, a purgative, and an emollient. The plant was not only dried and smoked, but its leaves were also applied locally to help heal wounds and burns, and powdered versions were swallowed to relieve mucus buildup in the throat. In California, desert tribes crushed tobacco leaves to create poultices to treat inflammatory diseases such as rheumatism, as well as skin infections such as eczema. The leaves were also smoked as a cure for the common cold, and were considered to be particularly effective if mixed with sage leaves. (And

now you've got an enjoyable alternative to downing a bottle of DayQuil
next winter.)

The "discovery" of the New
World was like an adrenaline shot
for European physicians, who practically tripped over themselves in their
excitement to uncover the healing
properties of the cornucopia of new
plants suddenly added to their medicine cabinets. Tobacco was one of the

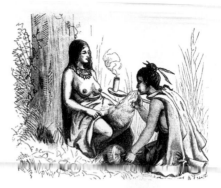

A Pawnee midwife uses medicinal tobacco on a woman in labor.

first champion New World crops warmly embraced by European doctors and
dubbed a panacea (although it certainly wasn't the last).

Spanish doctor Nicolás Monardes published a popular history of New
World medicinal plants in the 1570s, which included a glowing section on
tobacco. The book's euphoric title, *Joyful News Out of the New Found World*, says
a lot about the general feelings toward the new plant discoveries. Tobacco,
Monardes insisted, could cure upward of twenty diseases including cancer,
which is one of the most deeply ironic statements ever made in medical literature. (About seventeen people will die from smoking-induced lung cancer
in America in the next hour alone.)

THE RIGHT SNUFF: EARLY TOBACCO CHAMPIONS

Another early medical champion of tobacco was French ambassador to the
Portuguese court Jean Nicot, whose name was forever exalted in the annals of
medical literature as the origin of the word *nicotine*. (Nicotine is one of more
than four thousand chemicals generated when tobacco leaves are burned,
but it's the nastiest one in the bunch because it's what stimulates the brain
and nervous system of smokers, setting the stage for addiction.)

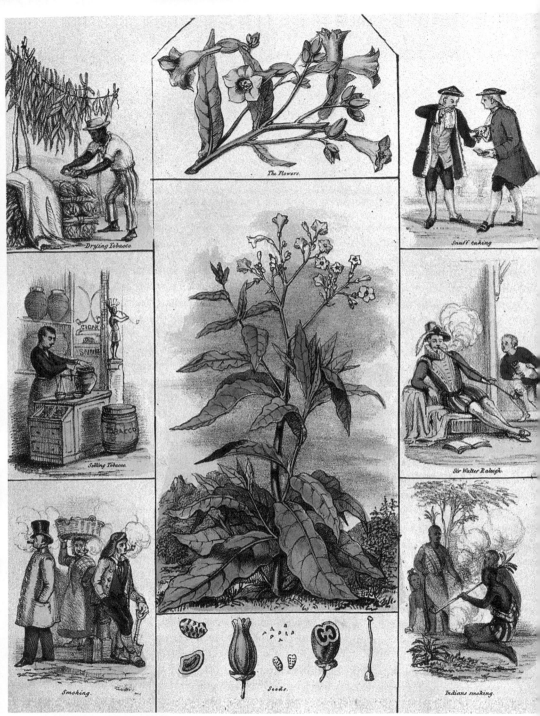

The Flowers.

Drying Tobacco.

Snuff taking

Selling Tobacco.

Sir Walter Raleigh.

Smoking.

Seeds.

Indians smoking.

The myriad wonders of the tobacco plant.

Nicot arrived in Lisbon in 1559, where he was quickly introduced to tobacco. A curious man with a scholarly bent, Nicot was deeply intrigued by this New World plant and early Portuguese experiments with its medical properties. The ambassador/budding physician decided to give it a go himself, so he whipped up a tobacco ointment, then nabbed a local man with a tumor and had the man apply the ointment regularly to his unwanted growth. (The local man's opinion in the matter has been lost to history.) The ointment worked, persuading Nicot that he was on the right track.

Convinced that tobacco was a nostrum and a potential cure for all manner of ills, Nicot bundled up some tobacco plants and made a triumphant return to France, where Catherine de' Medici was ruling as queen. In 1561, Nicot presented Catherine with tobacco plant leaves and instructions on how to powder the leaves and inhale them through her nose to relieve headaches. Catherine, who suffered from terrible headaches (poisoning all your enemies has that effect), took Nicot's advice. His tobacco snuff worked, making Catherine, and by extension the entirety of the French court, into an overnight tobacco convert.

As the French were setting just as many fashions in the sixteenth century as they are in the twenty-first, tobacco snuff quickly became de rigueur throughout the courts of Europe. There was hardly an aristocratic party you could attend in the late 1500s where someone wouldn't offer you a hit of the stuff. And it was only a matter of time before the fashionable drug made its way down the social strata and into the embrace of the masses. His fame and fortune secured, Nicot retired to the countryside and got to work on his next obsession: compiling a French dictionary.

In 1773, Swedish botanist Carl Linnaeus named the genus of tobacco cultivars *Nicotiana* in Nicot's honor, a nod to his role in popularizing the plant. It would be a dubious honor, however, once nicotine's seductive power was properly understood.

Despite Catherine de' Medici spreading the tobacco gospel, it wasn't all sunshine and roses for the plant, which had its naysayers in Europe from its early days of adoption. One of the most prominent anti-tobacco voices was that old killjoy King James I of England, who, writing in 1604, called tobacco smoking "loathsome." James went on, in a particularly prescient passage, to describe tobacco as "harmful to the brain, dangerous to the lungs."

James I's sentiments about tobacco began to catch on. As the seventeenth and eighteenth centuries progressed, the plant was no longer seen as a universal panacea. Tobacco smoke, however, was still recommended by some physicians for particular purposes. *Primitive Physick*, for example, a popular medical book from the mid-eighteenth through the mid-nineteenth centuries, recommended tobacco smoke—and this is one of our favorite remedies—to relieve earaches. If you suffered from an earache, all you had to do was grab a friend, and then have him light a pipe and blow the smoke deep into your ear canal. (Fun experiment: Try accompanying your coworker on his next cigarette break and asking for the same remedy.)

BLOWING SMOKE UP YOUR ARSE

Ear canals weren't the only body opening just waiting to receive a strong dose of secondhand smoke. You know the phrase "blowing smoke up your ass"? Well, you can disgust your next blind date with the true life medical origin of that phrase. Because literally blowing smoke up someone's ass was a sanctioned resuscitation method in the eighteenth century. The practice was so popular that tobacco smoke enema kits were manufactured and available for sale to concerned households. It's always best to be ready for a medical emergency and nothing says "prepared" like having a tobacco smoke enema kit next to your first aid supplies.

Tobacco smoke enemas had their day in the sun in the eighteenth century when they were embraced by the British medical community for a very particular purpose: the resuscitation of the drowned. These were the days when drowning in the River Thames was such a frequent occurrence that a society was actually formed and funded with the sole purpose of promoting the resuscitation of drowned people. Elaborately dubbed The Institution for Affording Immediate Relief to Persons Apparently Dead from Drowning, its members prowled the dangerous banks of the Thames, their tobacco smoke enema kits at the ready should any poor soul stumble into the river and need to be revived. If that happened, the society members would leap to the rescue, hauling the apparently drowned person out of the river, tearing off all of his clothes, rolling him onto his stomach, sticking an enema tube up his bottom, and striking up the fumigator and the bellows.

The bellows, by the way, were a welcome addition to the enema kit. Before the inclusion of bellows, you were stuck with blowing the smoke into someone's butt yourself. God forbid you accidentally inhaled. The results would not only be beyond disgusting but also potentially deadly. If your victim had cholera, for example, then you'd be a goner, too, by virtue of sucking

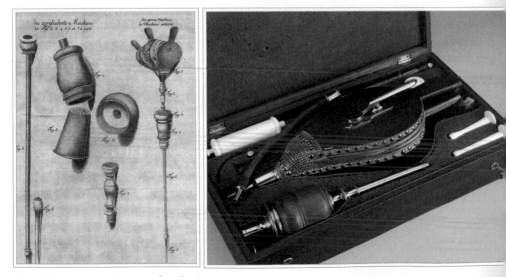

The smoke enema kit. No home is safe without one.

Remember not to inhale.

down cholera bacteria. And that, my friends, just about takes the cake for "worst way to die" featured in this book.

The medical thinking behind the kits seemed quite sound to its promoters, particularly Dr. William Hawes and Dr. Thomas Cogan, who founded the Thames rescue brigade. The smoke blown into the bodies of the apparently drowned was thought to accomplish two medical goals: warming the victim and stimulating respiration.

Of course, blowing smoke up someone's butt doesn't actually accomplish either of those goals, and that's why the phrase has been adopted today to mean an insincere compliment. It's a meaningless, pointless gesture. But it did give eighteenth-century rescuers a very . . . *intimate* view of a person's private area in an era when ankles were considered risqué, which probably explains some of the society's popularity.

If the smoke enema didn't revive the victim, the institution members turned to a much more reliable method that actually saved lives: artificial respiration. Mouth-to-mouth rescue breathing, however, was largely frowned upon by the medical community as "vulgar," as compared, say, to blowing smoke up someone's butt. Would-be resuscitators used bellows to pump air into the lungs of the nearly drowned. Midwives, however, knew better and regularly practiced mouth-to-mouth rescue breathing to resuscitate infants. Thankfully, the rest of the medical community eventually caught up with the midwives, mouth-to-mouth lost its "vulgar" connotation, and countless lives were saved as a result.

Smoke a Cigarette, Clean Your House!

Although tobacco smoke enemas were never a good idea, tobacco did have a brief run as a disinfectant, an intriguing use of its smoke that may not be ineffective. Columbus's crew had observed the Taíno people of Cuba using burning tobacco leaves to disinfect homes where people had been sick, and its reputation as a disinfectant migrated with the plant to Europe.

During a plague outbreak in London in 1665, schoolchildren were actually told to smoke in their classrooms as a way to ward off the disease. In what was possibly the only upside to being alive in London during a plague outbreak, the schoolchildren didn't have to play hooky to get their nicotine fix.

Similarly, in 1882, in an outbreak of smallpox in Bolton, all the residents of a particular workhouse were issued tobacco to help keep the establishment free of germs.

Tobacco's potential as a disinfectant was only occasionally examined by physicians. In 1889, an anonymous author writing in the *British Medical Journal* mentioned that the compound pyridine, present in tobacco smoke, kills germs and in turn appears to lower the risk of tobacco smokers to infectious diseases such as diphtheria and typhus. In 1913, an article in *The Lancet* further examined pyridine in tobacco smoke, again demonstrating that tobacco smoke killed the bacterium causing cholera.

Both articles, however, were also quick to mention that the harmful effects of smoking tobacco outweighed its potential benefits, an argument that has largely halted any further investigation into tobacco's potential use as a disinfectant.

TOBACCO TOOTHPASTE

Some American Indian tribes combined powdered tobacco with lime or chalk to create a sort of toothpaste for teeth cleaning, a potential benefit not enjoyed by today's tobacco users, who frequently have stained teeth from chewing or smoking tobacco.

Tobacco toothpaste is still in use in South Asia, where companies such as IPCO market it commercially. IPCO's toothpaste, Creamy Snuff, in addition to having the best toothpaste name ever created (take that, Colgate), contains clove oil, glycerin, spearmint, menthol, camphor, and, of course, tobacco. Creamy Snuff is particularly popular among South Asian women, some of whom use the toothpaste eight to ten times per day under encouragement from the manufacturer to "let it linger" in their mouths. (The tobacco in Creamy Snuff is not the only entry, by the way, in the competition for Worst Toothpaste Ingredient found in this book. Check out the radioactive toothpaste profiled in the Radium & Radon chapter for another competitor.)

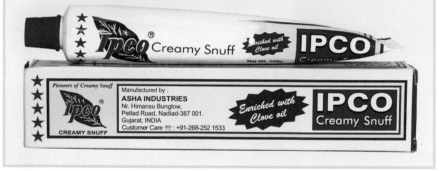

THE TOBACCO INDUSTRY
BEDS DOWN WITH PHYSICIANS

The nineteenth century seemed like the beginning of the end for medicinal tobacco. In 1811, English scientist Ben Brodie discovered that nicotine was harmful to the heart. In 1828, researchers went on to isolate the nicotine alkaloid, a discovery that further lowered medical opinion of the plant, as the negative impact of nicotine on the brain and nervous system could now be observed.

By the early twentieth century, concerns began to surface about the health risks of cigarette smoking. An alarmed tobacco industry, in an effort to allay consumer fears, forged a powerful alliance with physicians. Doctors, who smoked almost as frequently as the general public, were still digesting the recent crop of research indicating potential health risks of smoking with the curious fact that not everyone who smokes ends up sick. It wasn't terribly

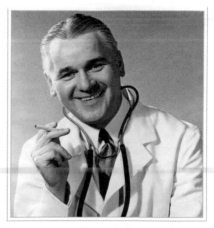

"More Doctors smoke Camels than any other cigarette!"

difficult, therefore, to find physicians willing to offer testimonials for tobacco companies, especially when they were offered cases of cigarettes to feed their own habits in exchange for their support.

Starting with a successful American Tobacco Company campaign that advertised Lucky Strikes as being "less irritating," physicians began cropping up in colorful ads in magazines promoting cigarettes. In the 1930s, Philip Morris, a newcomer to the game, made a name for itself with a large and successful advertising campaign reporting that a "group of doctors" found its cigarettes to improve or completely clear irritation of the nose and throat from smoking. The campaign almost single-handedly made Philip Morris into a major brand.

The doctors-with-cigarettes advertising frenzy came to a head with the "More doctors smoke Camels than any other cigarette" campaign launched by the R. J. Reynolds Tobacco Company. Between 1946 and 1952, Camel advertisements were led by this slogan generated from an "independent survey." The survey, as it turned out, was actually conducted by the William Esty Co., an R. J. Reynolds subsidiary, which questioned physicians about their favorite cigarette brand after providing them with complimentary cartons of Camel cigarettes.

Tobacco Today

The "More doctors . . ." campaign was the beginning of the end. As more and more studies surfaced showing the harmful effects of cigarette smoking, tobacco was on its way out the medical door. Physicians transitioned from using tobacco in treatments to understanding, and then combating, the numerous ill-effects of smoking (cancer, emphysema, heart disease, asthma, and diabetes, to name a few).

In the meantime, however, we had embraced recreational tobacco smoking on a global scale. Even though the harmful effects of smoking have been well understood and heavily promoted for decades, there are still 1.3 billion people around the world who smoke cigarettes regularly, and the global tobacco industry is a $300 billion juggernaut. So physicians have been understandably a bit too busy fighting the negative impacts of smoking on the human body to further experiment with any positive properties of tobacco.

And happily for modern-day walkers along the River Thames, tobacco smoke enemas are no longer the preferred resuscitation method for the nearly drowned. We can all feel a bit safer when visiting the Thames knowing there's not a creepster waiting in the wings to blow tobacco smoke up our bums if we should fall in.

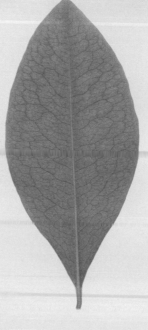

9

Cocaine

Euphoric Cocaine Experiments, Sigmund Freud, Cocaine Toothache Drops, Vin Mariani, and a Dying President

A week after Robert E. Lee surrendered to Ulysses S. Grant, one of the last battles of the Civil War was fought on the Chattahoochee River separating Alabama and Georgia. Few things in life are as deeply ironic as being forced to participate in a battle after a war has effectively ended. Thanks to glacially slow communication lines, however, the Battle of Columbus happened a full week after Lee had surrendered his troops at Appomattox Courthouse.

At the battle, a thirty-four-year-old Confederate lieutenant colonel named John Pemberton very nearly lost his life during a cavalry charge. Pemberton took a nasty saber wound to his chest that could have easily killed him, but thankfully for him and for future soda enthusiasts, he lived.

While recovering from his wounds, Pemberton, like many of his comrades on both sides of the Civil War, became addicted to morphine. Unlike many of his fellow wounded soldiers, however, Pemberton was a pharmacist in his civilian life. As such, he had access to a variety of drugs and herbal supplements with which he could experiment. (And experiment he did, concocting a variety of patent medicines such as Botanic Blood Balm, Tripex Liver Pills, Globe Flower Cough Syrup, and Indian Queen Hair Dye.) After recovering, he was determined to find—and patent—an alternative painkiller to morphine. Something a little less, you know, opiate-y.

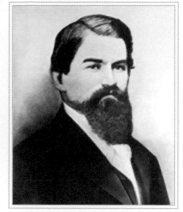

Above: Lt. Col. John Pemberton, plus beard. Below: An innocent coca shrub, perfect for your backyard.

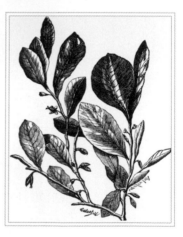

Pemberton started by extracting cocaine from coca, an ancient plant popular in South America and recently embraced in France as a stimulant and cure-all in the form of coca wine (more on that later). Soon he had concocted a homegrown American alternative to French coca wine, an alcoholic, cocaine-laced drink that he took to Atlanta to sell.

That buzzy little drink he patented was called Coca-Cola.

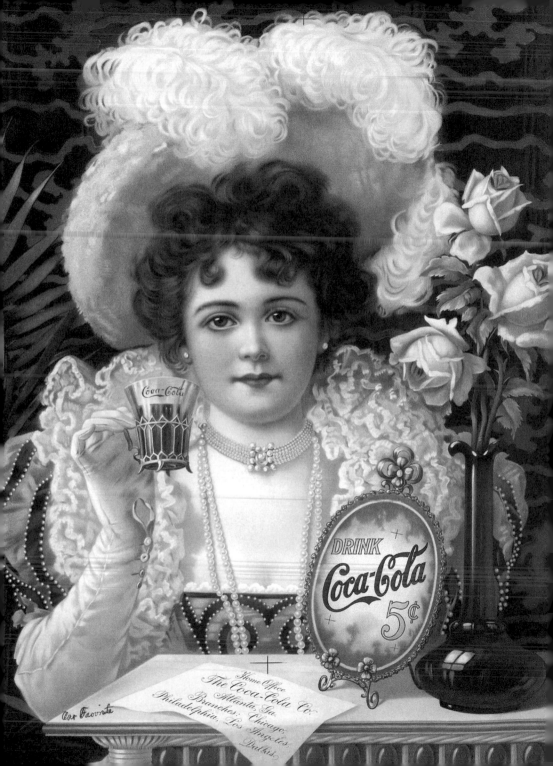

NATURE'S STIMULANT:
FROM THE ANDES TO AUSTRIA

Cocaine—"the caviar of street drugs" and one of the most popular recreational drugs on the planet—has been employed as a stimulant since at least 3000 BCE. Cocaine is derived from the *Erythroxylum coca* plant, native to the Andean mountains of South America. The plant looks decidedly normal, almost innocent, just another shrub in a sea of shrubby plants. But that little shrub, which wouldn't look out of place in your landscaped yard, has made countless fortunes and ruined countless lives.

The leaves of the coca plant were widely chewed by the Inca in Peru for their stimulative effect, a practice that was summarily banned by Spain's Catholic Church after the arrival of the conquistadores in the sixteenth century.

Their plan, however, didn't work out very well. Frequent and large-scale use of coca leaves eventually forced the Spanish colonial government to concede defeat. As one conquistador wrote in 1539:

> Coca, which is the leaf of a small tree that resembles the sumac
> found in our own Castile, is one thing that the Indians are ne'er
> without in their mouths, that they say sustains them and gives
> them refreshment, so that, even under the sun they feel not the
> heat, and it is worth its weight in gold in these parts, accounting for
> the major portion of the tithes.

Coca use was endemic. Eventually, the Spanish just said screw it and started getting high on the leaves themselves. They also began to tax and regulate its sale and use, an intelligent strategy of narcotic governance.

Conquistadores also brought coca leaves back with them to Europe, where they were almost totally ignored because of all the shiny gold and silver that was loading down their ships. It didn't help that if any coca leaves in a bunch get moist, the whole batch will quickly rot, which was a particular challenge for ship transport. So it took a while for the rest of Europe to start investigating those funny leaves from South America.

As the science of alkaloid extraction advanced in the early nineteenth century, however, it was inevitable that someone would eventually turn their attention to the leaves of the coca shrub. In 1859, a large quantity made its way to Germany and into the hands of a bright young doctoral student named Albert Niemann, who was in need of a thesis. The graduate student decided to try extracting the active ingredient from coca leaves. He succeeded, isolating cocaine and earning his doctorate degree in one fell swoop, all the while becoming the first and last person to earn an advanced degree for creating a highly addictive recreational drug. (And if creating cocaine wasn't a terrible enough legacy, the twenty-six-year-old doctor began experimenting with ethylene and sulfur dichloride, eventually inventing mustard gas and killing himself in the process.)

The same year that Niemann was extracting cocaine, an Italian doctor named Paolo Mantegazza also became enamored of the coca plant, traveling to Peru and enthusiastically volunteering himself as a lab rat for testing the effects of coca leaf doses. Not one to shy away from extremes, Mantegazza diligently recorded his reaction to small, moderate, high, and ridiculously high doses of coca leaves. He noticed his reduced hunger and improved energy on small and moderate doses and commented happily on the "rush" he received from large doses, writing:

> I sneered at the poor mortals condemned to live in this valley of tears while I, carried on the wings of two leaves of coca, went flying through the spaces of 77,438 words, each more splendid than the one before. . . . God is unjust because he made man incapable of sustaining the effects of coca all life long. I would rather live a life of ten years with coca than one of 100,000 (and here I inserted a line of zeroes) without it.

Such enthusiasm, published by Mantegazza in his pamphlet "On the Hygienic and Medical Values of Coca," did not go unnoticed by the European populace. And he's right, cocaine does make its user feel supremely confident, decisive, and full of energy—all of which are useful traits for many professions.

It's no surprise that cocaine use became popular among intellectuals, artists, writers, and other people who relied upon a highly functioning brain for their work output. The most famous advocate of cocaine as a stimulant in the nineteenth century was none other than Sigmund Freud, who became an all-out addict in his twenties and thirties. Freud wrote to a colleague in 1895 after "a cocainization of the left nostril," that "in the last few days I have felt unbelievably well, as though everything had been erased. . . . I have felt wonderful, as though there had never been anything wrong at all." Freud quit by the time he was forty, before he wrote the major works of psychology that have turned him into a household name. Scholars still debate, however, the long-term impact of Freud's cocaine addiction on the brilliance of his later ideas.

No More Pain with Cocaine

The young Freud championed the use of cocaine not only as a stimulant, but also as a local anesthetic, something else it's actually quite good at. He passed on his knowledge to the ophthalmologist Karl Koller, who used cocaine as a topical anesthetic during eye surgery to great success, his results published in the British medical journal *The Lancet*.

A young American doctor named William Stewart Halsted (noted for founding Johns Hopkins Hospital and pioneering the radical mastectomy) read about Koller's experiments and gave them a try himself, employing cocaine to numb the pain of dental surgery and practicing the technique on his graduate students (we're sure they thanked him for the privilege).

Naturally, cocaine's pain-relieving skills led to its enthusiastic embrace by the burgeoning producers of patent medicines in the late nineteenth and early twentieth centuries. Cocaine was a major ingredient in many popular medications, including Roger's Cocaine Pile Remedy and Lloyd's Cocaine Toothache Drops. (Consumers were assured that these products did not, in fact, contain any addictive drugs. *cough*)

Roger's Cocaine Pile Remedy was intended to shrink large and painful hemorrhoids. The pill, taken as a suppository, was probably somewhat effective because cocaine does have the ability to shrink inflamed tissue.

Lloyd's Cocaine Toothache Drops—advertised as an "instantaneous cure!"—were likely invented in the wake of Dr. Halsted's successful experiments with cocaine in dental surgery. At the cost of $0.15 a package, the toothache drops were quite affordable. They were also proudly marketed for use with children.

The terribly tragic outcome of Halsted's experiments with cocaine was his own addiction. The doctor began injecting cocaine directly into his veins for its stimulative effects, quickly becoming an addict. Eventually, he was sent to Butler Hospital in Providence, Rhode Island, where the recognized treatment for drug addiction was injecting the patient with large doses of morphine.

Halsted eventually left the sanatorium a broken man, crippled with addictions to both morphine and cocaine. Not that he let that stop him from practicing medicine.

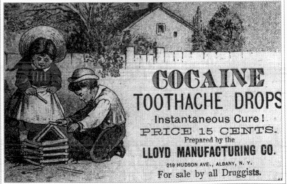

The sweet innocence of a bygone age.

DR. JEKYLL AND MR. HYDE

There is some evidence to suggest that Robert Louis Stevenson wrote *Dr. Jekyll and Mr. Hyde* while on a six-day cocaine binge; indeed, to some readers, the story read like a metaphor for cocaine addiction itself. (Guess which version of the protagonist symbolizes the addict.) Oscar Wilde wrote of the novella, "The transformation of Dr. Jekyll reads dangerously like an experiment out of *The Lancet*." A *JAMA* article in 1971 closely examined this allegation, noting that at the

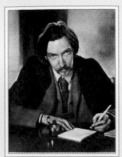

time of writing, Stevenson was basically an invalid, confined by his doctor to bedrest and under strict instructions not to even speak for fear of upsetting his "pulmonary hemorrhages." Yet, despite this, Stevenson wrote the novella in an astonishingly short period of time, wherein he didn't even stop to eat or sleep for six days. That fact, combined with the nature of the novella itself, makes for a pretty convincing case that Stevenson was high as a kite on cocaine during its composition.

BOTTOMS UP:
ADVENTURES IN DRINKABLE COCAINE

As cocaine was embraced by the patent medicine community, cocaine-based tonics started popping up everywhere. Take the invitingly named Coca Beef Tonic, which was meant to be a substitute for meat. If you couldn't afford a nice slice of filet mignon, you could instead cough up a few pennies for a beef-flavored beverage. The tonic made up for the lack of meat in your diet by containing cocaine and 23 percent alcohol. Few things combat hunger as well as getting mind-blowingly drunk and high at the same time.

A far more popular method of cocaine distribution, however, was in wine. Angelo Mariani, a French chemist who read about Mantegazza's euphoric self-experimentation with coca leaves, decided to toss a few leaves in a good bottle of Bordeaux and see what happened next. The ethanol in the wine extracted

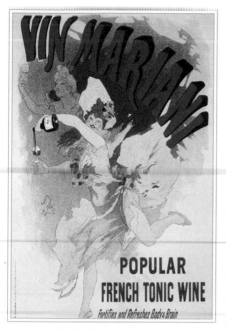

Cocaine dissolved in alcohol!
"Fortifies and Refreshes Body & Brain."

the cocaine from the coca leaves, which then dissolved and made for one heady drink. Mariani, pleased with the effect, starting bottling up Bordeaux with coca leaves, called the product Vin Mariani, advertised the concoction as a tonic wine, and sat back to reap a fortune. Because, shockingly, Vin Mariani was a hit. At 10 percent alcohol and 8 percent cocaine extract, how could it be anything else? Vin Mariani was so popular that it made the French chemist into a multimillionaire, perhaps the first major fortune founded on blow.

The drink also attracted a wide range of celebrity endorsements and was partially responsible for a substantial degree of late-nineteenth-century literary output: Arthur Conan Doyle, Jules Verne, Alexandre Dumas, Henrik Ibsen, and Robert Louis Stevenson were all dedicated and enthusiastic drinkers, a fact worth remembering the next time you're stumbling through overly long late-nineteenth-century classics. Cocaine, remember, makes a user supremely confident in their decisions, and, in the case of a novelist, less inclined to edit.

Queen Victoria was a fan of Vin Mariani, as were Popes Leo XIII and Pius X. Thomas Edison drank the wine because it helped to keep him awake during his all-night experiments with electricity. (The committed genius slept only four hours a night. He really needed this stuff.) And former President Ulysses S. Grant, dying slowly from throat cancer, downed bottle after bottle of Vin Mariani to dull the pain as he completed his memoirs.

Vin Mariani was all the rage. And products that are all the rage tend to attract competitors. Competitors, for example, like John Pemberton's French Wine Coca, eventually shortened to Coca-Cola. When Coca-Cola was first sold on the market in 1886, we know it contained cocaine. What we don't know—and what no one alive now knows—is how much. (The authors are inclined to think it contained quite a bit.) The drink was advertised as a "brain tonic and intellectual beverage" and was credited with easing menstrual cramps. By 1905, it was found to contain $1/400$th of a grain of cocaine per ounce of syrup. And by 1929, Coca-Cola was officially cocaine free. (The *cola* part of the name, by the way, comes from another ingredient in the mix: the extract of African kola nuts, which contain caffeine and are chewed in West Africa to produce a mild stimulative effect.)

Drink Your Coke, Participate in History

Today, Coca-Cola still actually contains coca extract, just without the fun part. Although the exact recipe is a closely guarded trade secret, the company does import coca leaves legally from Peru's National Coca Company. After the cocaine is extracted and sold for pharmaceutical use by eye, ear, nose, and throat specialists as a topical anesthesia, the remaining flavor of the coca leaves is enveloped into the secret recipe.

So, although you can't legally drink cocaine-laced wine anymore, it's nice to know that a refreshing glass of ice-cold Coca-Cola—the greatest success story in the history of beverages—still has a hint of coca leaves in its taste. That little touch of history in every can of Coke connects you with a five-thousand-year-old story of humans getting high on cocaine.

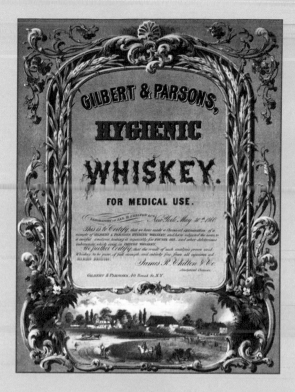

10

Alcohol

Of Cavemen, Disemboweled Gladiators, the Black Plague, Drunken Wet-Nurses, and Brandy Injections

For thousands of years, mankind struggled through its existence, just trying to kill enough mammoths to get through the week with maybe a relaxing fire to look forward to on the weekend. Then, on some glorious day lost to the mists of time, a Neolithic caveman accidentally left out an earthen jar with some berry juice in it for a few days. And so alcohol was discovered, and mankind suddenly had a new reason to get up in the morning.

Ever since that auspicious day, alcohol—specifically ethanol—has been a staple in our diet and our medicine cabinet. Early humans, in addition to noticing the pleasing impact of alcohol on the brain, realized that it was an effective antiseptic when applied to wounds and slightly anesthetic when you had to get those wounds stitched back together again.

"Did little Billy get mauled by a saber-toothed tiger again? Let's grab the berry wine."

It wasn't long before humans realized that alcohol was also an excellent solvent, particularly good at extracting active ingredients from herbs. And so the seeds were sown to unite medicine and alcohol throughout history. Here are some of the stops along the way between the Neolithic caveman's fermented berry juice and today's after-work glass of wine.

WINE

When humans were still a few millennia away from figuring out distillation, wine was the alcohol of choice for medicinal concoctions. Really, the only choice. So ancient remedies, from Egypt to Greece to Rome, all recommended infusing herbs in wine for a multitude of ailments.

But it was ancient Rome that really perfected the art of winemaking and loudly proclaimed its health benefits. Depression, memory problems, grief? Drink some wine. Bloating, constipation, urinary problems, diarrhea, gout? Drink some more wine. Snakebites? Tapeworms? Let's get smashed.

One recipe, described by Cato, was for a wine infusion to help with constipation: treat grapevines with a mixture of ashes, manure, and hellebore (a deeply poisonous plant). Can you imagine the sommelier's description?

"Lightly fruity, with hints of ash, manure, and poison."

Cato went on to suggest that urinary troubles could be cured by mixing old wine with juniper berries and boiling them in a lead pot. The lead poisoning and saturnine gout were added bonuses.

Galen, briefly responsible for the medical care of gladiators in Pergamon, liberally used wine to disinfect wounds—including soaking the bowels of severely wounded gladiators in wine before placing them back inside their bodies. (One extreme way of getting drunk not yet embraced by American fraternities.)

It wasn't all just one big Bacchanalia, however, and some Roman writers described the negative impacts of drinking too much wine, which they felt magnified the personality defects of the drinker. Public drunkenness was frowned upon during official functions, such as the Senate, where Mark Antony once was so hungover that he vomited.

Wine's reputation as a healer followed it out of Rome and into the Dark Ages in Europe, where monasteries kept up the tradition of using wine as medicine. The thirteenth-century friar Roger Bacon wrote that wine could "preserve the stomach, strengthen the natural heat, help digestion, defend the body from corruption, concoct the food till it be turned into very blood."

Bacon, however, also cautioned against overindulgence in wine:

Bacchus toasts to your health.

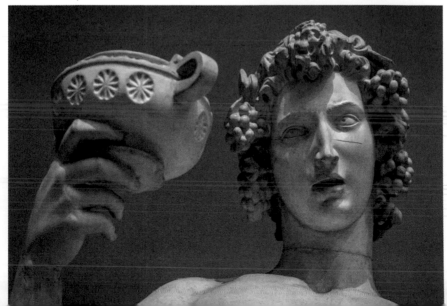

If it be over-much guzzled, it will on the contrary do a great deal of harm: For it will darken the understanding, ill-affect the brain, render the natural vigor languid, bring forgetfulness, weaken the joints, beget shaking of the limbs and bleareyedness; it will darken and make black the blood of the heart, whence fear, trembling, and many diseases arise.

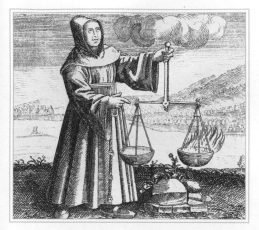

Roger Bacon at work. Job perk for medieval scientists: cool robes.

Sounds like Bacon was no stranger to drunkenness.

Wine kept its place in the medicinal arsenal all the way up to the twentieth century, where it struggled a bit (Prohibition was rough), but it has enjoyed a recent revival in the medical field, where the oft-repeated recommendation of a glass of red wine per day has been suggested to reduce the risk of heart disease.

GIN

Juniper berries have enjoyed a long association with healing. In ancient Egypt, they were thought to cure jaundice. In ancient Greece, they were prescribed for colic and as a little performance booster before those naked wrestling matches. The berries finally made their way into alcoholic concoctions in ancient Rome, where Dioscorides prescribed juniper berries steeped in wine to help cure chest pains.

In the first century, Pliny the Elder also wrote about the health benefits of infusing alcohol with juniper berries, although in his case he noted that steeping berries in red wine would "act astringently on the bowels."

The astringency of juniper, however, made it a favorite with physicians, and by the time the Black Plague swept its way through Europe, taking an estimated 100 million lives with it, physicians recommended patients burn juniper incense, rub juniper oil on their bodies, wear plague masks complete with juniper berries stuffed in them, and drink juniper cordials to fumigate their bodies and strengthen their constitutions.

It just so happened that around the same time that the Black Plague reached its height (**mid-fourteenth century**), Dutch distillers were experimenting with making brandy. Perhaps the desperation of the plague-stricken populace led those distillers to try tossing juniper berries into their concoctions as a potential protection (bonus!) to go with the brandy.

Quickly moving on from brandy, which relied upon grapes (not particularly easy to grow in Holland's northern climate), the Dutch began experimenting with alcohol distilled from grain, all the while keeping the juniper berries as added ingredients.

And so proto-gin was born. The Dutch quickly worked these juniper drinks into their medical cabinets, where they were drunk for quite a few different purposes. Nursing mothers and wet nurses even drank gin to pass some of the healing properties of juniper on to the infants in their care. According to William Worth, a Dutch-English distiller:

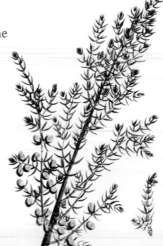

Juniper berries en route to becoming something awesome.

> It is a general custom in Holland, when the
> Child is troubled with Oppressions of
> Wind, for the Mother whilst the Child
> is sucking, to drink of the Powers or
> Spirits of Juniper, by which the Child is
> Relieved.

By the fifteenth century, most Dutch towns had their own distiller churning out this particular alcoholic invention, which they called *genever*. Although its initial origins were medical, gin quickly became favored throughout northern Europe for its taste and pleasing impacts on the mind.

When genever made its way over to England, the working-class British, used to drinking watered-down beer, were quite literally floored by the high alcoholic content of the beverage. And so began the gin craze of the early eighteenth century, which would go on to ruin a staggering number of lives, and, in the process, transition gin firmly out of the medicine cabinet and into the gin shop.

Today, we now know that overconsumption of gin—or really any alcohol—can also lead to "gin blossoms." Yes, sometimes that means a late-night dose of sentimentality and "Hey Jealousy" on repeat as you wax nostalgic about the Clinton years, but also, more harmfully, gin blossoms on your face. These gin blossoms are the red lines and dots on the faces of heavy drinkers, which are dilated capillaries caused by drinking too much alcohol.

WILLIAM THE CONQUEROR'S EXPLODING CORPSE

William the Conqueror (1028–1087) wasn't really feeling the "conqueror" part of his name as he advanced in years and his weight caught up with him. When William had grown so fat that he was having difficulty riding, he decided it was time to conquer his own body. With a diet. A hardcore diet consisting of nothing but alcohol. William lay in bed and basically went on a lengthy bender. And it worked. He soon lost enough weight to ride horses again, an irony, it turned out, because riding horses led to his untimely death. In 1087, William's belly (still quite corpulent), smashed into the pommel of his saddle with so much force that it caused internal damage. William eventually died from the wound. In a horrifying historical side note to categorize under "how the mighty have fallen," William's already bloating body proved too large for his previously arranged sarcophagus. When his attendants attempted to force his body into the coffin, the body literally popped, filling the church with a terrible stench and a variety of disgusting bodily fluids. Needless to say, it was a brief funeral.

BRANDY

Brandy is so universally regarded as superior to all other spirits
from a medicinal point of view . . .

—*The Lancet,* 1902

Before the arrival of the Moors in
southern Europe in the eighth century,
Europe was strictly a place for wine
and beer. The North Africans, in addition to reintroducing Europe to science
and mathematics, brought with them
the fine art of distillation. In a quest for
new medicines, the Moors tried distilling almost anything they could get their
hands on— including the local wines
in Spain, where they had made their
strongholds.

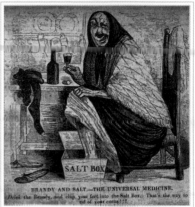

*Brandy and salt: the universal panacea.
Don't you want to look like her?*

When you distill wine down to its essence, you get a highly concentrated liquor, which today we call brandy. When the Spanish reclaimed the
Iberian peninsula, the Moors left behind their distillation practices and a
local taste for this new alcoholic beverage. Spanish monasteries kept up the
tradition of distilling wine into brandy and began shipping it around the
Christian world, including to the Vatican, where the papal doctor began
prescribing it as a life-prolonging tonic. Soon brandy caught on as a health
drink in its own right.

For the next few hundred years, brandy enjoyed the greatest praise of
all the alcoholic drinks in the medical world. It was considered a stimulant and was often the first item turned to in the case of fainting. *Did Lady
Arabella swoon and faint at your dashing entrance? Revive her with a shot of
brandy.*

THE MYTH OF KEG-CARRYING ST. BERNARDS

St. Bernard dogs were kept at a monastery on the remote and dangerous St. Bernard's Pass in the Alps, on hand to help with search-and-rescue missions for the many travelers stranded by snowstorms or avalanches. The dogs were extremely good at this job, able to sniff out humans and keep them warm until help could arrive. According to popular legend, the St. Bernards also carried alcohol in kegs around their necks to help warm and revive the hypothermic people they encountered. Athough it's a pleasant story—and really, the sight of a warm dog and a keg of alcohol would rally the spirit if you were stranded in a snowstorm—it's pure legend. No historical document survives recording this practice. Which is probably for the best, considering the impact of alcohol on hypothermic patients.

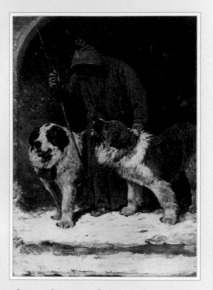

A historical painting of a historical inaccuracy.

Physicians also utilized brandy when faced with hemorrhaging patients because alcohol was thought to promote clotting. Brandy was even sometimes injected directly into a patient's arm, up his bum, or intravenously during a difficult pregnancy. It's easy to imagine mothers in the agonies of childbirth in days before epidurals shouting "Just give me the damn brandy injection!"

Brandy was also thought to work as a stimulant in cases of hypothermia, a reputation that made brandy a critical part of the supplies for early explorations of the Arctic. The problem is that although alcohol makes you *feel* warmer, it actually contributes to heat loss by widening your blood vessels at first. Later, it can tighten vessels and exacerbate frostbite. Nevertheless, even today, when this biological process is better understood, you'll still find hunters in cold climates with a flask of alcohol in their bag of supplies. They are combining two terrible ideas in one horrendous package: Mixing guns and alcohol, and drinking to "stay warm."

Although the vasoactive effect of alcohol makes it a poor choice for hypothermic cases, gram for gram, alcohol supplies more calories than protein or carbohydrates. That fact, combined with its tendency to calm sick patients by intoxicating them, led many nineteenth-century doctors to include alcohol in their medical arsenal.

Even as recently as the early 1900s, physicians were still prescribing brandy as a general health tonic. By the end of World War I, though, as pathology was better understood and new intravenous concoctions appeared, brandy fell from its honored place on the physician's shelf.

BEER

Despite being around for possibly longer than wine, beer has never quite enjoyed the same medical reputation. Even the doctors of yore seemed to recognize that the drawbacks outweighed the benefits. According to Italian physician Aldobrandino of Siena in 1256:

> But from whichever it is made, whether from oats, barley or wheat,
> it harms the head and the stomach, it causes bad breath and ruins
> the teeth, it fills the stomach with bad fumes, and as a result anyone
> who drinks it along with wine becomes drunk quickly; but it does
> have the property of facilitating urination and makes one's flesh
> white and smooth.

Aldobrandino does have a good point about beer facilitating urination. Just ask the guy walking around downtown on a Friday night with that urgent look in his eyes.

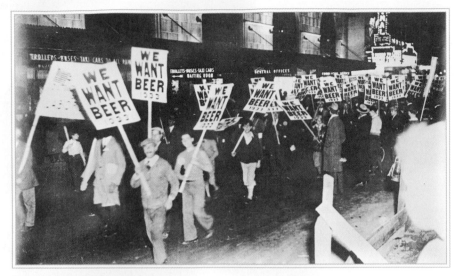

Literally the best protest signs of all time.

Medicinal beer as a concept did crop up, somewhat bizarrely, during Prohibition, when a handful of special interest groups united around the common cause of making alcohol—really just any kind of alcohol—available for medical purchase. Having given up on anything harder than wine or beer, advocates began promoting the medicinal benefits of beer in the hopes that an exception to the Volstead Act (passed in 1919 to ban the consumption of alcohol) might be forthcoming from the government. Although medicinal beer would eventually earn a place in present-day hospitals, where doctors sometimes prescribe beer to patients to prevent withdrawal, Prohibition-era alcoholics weren't so fortunate.

"Since Prohibition went into effect I have been approached by a number of physicians who appealed to me for beer on the ground that it was absolutely necessary for the welfare of their patients," said Colonel Jacob Ruppert, a brewer who also happened to own the New York Yankees. Ruppert sadly informed the *New York Times* that he "was not in a position to help them."

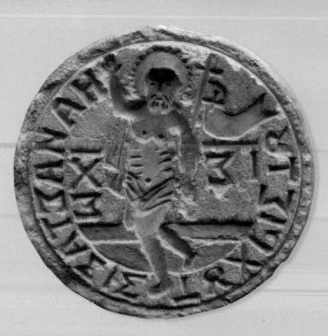

11

Earth

Of Death Row Deals, Terra Sigillata, Traveling Miners, Poisoning Dogs, and Dirt-Eaters

In 1581, young Wendel Thumblardt's days were numbered. Condemned in the town of Hohenlohe, Germany, for a string of robberies, Thumblardt was sentenced to the gallows. He had one more card up his sleeve, though. He'd heard of a powerful poison antidote called terra sigillata, or "sealed earth," just then making its way around Germany. He proposed that instead of hanging him, they use his body like a lab rat.

Thumblardt suggested they poison him with "the most deadly poison that might be devised." And then a "perfit trial might bee had of the worthiness of this medicinable earth." It was a clever wager: If he died, well, that's where he was heading anyway. But if he lived, he would walk a free man.

Wolfgang II, prince of the district, was sufficiently intrigued. Just several days before, a German-miner-turned-traveling-physician named Andreas Berthold had shown up in town, peddling little clay tablets known as terra sigillata. According to Berthold, these tablets were a panacea for just about anything that ailed you, but their special ability was to serve as an antidote to poison. Antidotes were a big deal at the time, when poisoning someone was as easy as a trip to your local apothecary, a quick dash of some powder in a wineglass, and Bob's your uncle. Like any good ruler in the sixteenth century, when the Medicis were in power all over Europe, Wolfgang II took poison antidotes seriously.

He agreed to the criminal's request.

Thumblardt was dragged up from some hellish dungeon and forced to ingest a dram and a half of "mercury sublimate, mingled with conserve of roses." The prisoner truly got his wish of receiving "the most deadly poison that might be devised." Mercury poisoning is a vicious, terrible way to die, complete with horrendous renal damage and the deeply painful corrosion of your mucus membranes and stomach lining . . . while you are still conscious. The amount they forced on the criminal, thoughtfully combined with a rose conserve to make it go down easier, was three times the dose needed to kill someone.

Wolfgang II wasn't taking any chances.

After downing his poison, Thumblardt was immediately given some wine into which 4 grams of Berthold's terra sigillata tablets had been dissolved.

Lo and behold, Thumblardt survived to see another day, although not before "the poison did extremely torment and vexe him." Figuring that surviving mercury poisoning was probably a sufficient theft deterrent,

Wolfgang II made it his first order of business to release Thumblardt into the care of his parents. His second move was to buy a lifetime supply of terra sigillata from the traveling salesman. He even gave Berthold a letter bearing his stamp of approval so he could safely move around Germany advertising his tablets of earth.

ANCIENT EARTH, SACRED EARTH

The practice of geophagy—that is, eating dirt—is considerably ancient, going back to at least 500 BCE, when the inhabitants of Lemnos, a Grecian island in the Mediterranean, harvested red medicinal clay from a particular hill on a special day each year. With government officials supervising the process, the clay

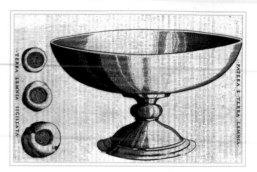

Terra sigillata from Lemnos, overshadowed by a large cup.

was washed, refined, rolled to a particular thickness, and then formed into little tablets. The island's priestesses stepped in next, blessing and stamping the tablets with their official seal (hence the name terra sigillata, meaning "sealed earth") before distributing them to the Lemnos equivalent of pharmacies, where the clay was sold as a medicinal aid.

For what? you might ask. Clay has been used as an antidote since antiquity, as it slows down absorbtion of drugs within the digestive tract. It's even helpful for healing wounds. The quackery part comes from the religious significance awarded the little clay tablets, the special geographic focus claimed to enhance their power, and the cure-all capabilites assigned to them. Clay can be effective in certain medical situations, even if it's not blessed and stamped by a priestess or dug from the hills of Lemnos.

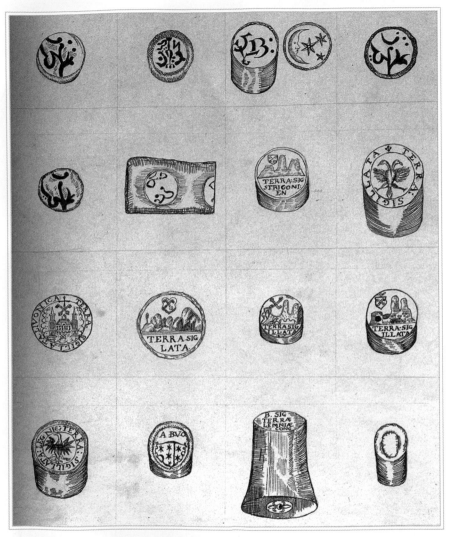

Various seals for terra sigillatas around Europe. Collect them all!

Hippocrates himself mentions the healing properties of ingesting clay tablets, in his case referencing clay from the island of Samos. He was followed by Dioscorides, who recommended clay as an antidote, an astringent, and an antidiarrheal, and Galen, who traveled to Lemnos to watch the production of terra

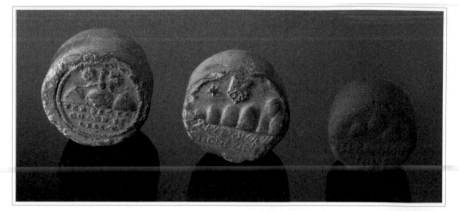

Quick, you've just been poisoned and have three choices for your terra sigillata antidote: silver, gold, or red.

sigillata in person. He was impressed. So impressed that he took back twenty thousand tablets to Rome in 167 CE.

Terra sigillata distribution waned with the fall of the Classical world, not appearing again until it made its way back into Europe via the invading forces of the Ottoman Turks, who were convinced that a special clay from Armenia was a cure for the plague. Although ingesting Armenian clay would have been technically ineffective against the bacterial onslaught of the bubonic plague, the placebo effect of ingesting something sacred or special may indeed have contributed to the occasional recovery.

One area the Turks occupied? The land around Striga (present-day Strzegom, Poland), where Andreas Berthold lived and worked as a miner.

BUILDING AN EMPIRE OUT OF CLAY

Berthold had shown up in several towns in Germany, advertising his terra sigillata to the local leaders. In his wake, he left a string of dead dogs, who were the lab animal of choice when the townsfolk wanted to see if the mysterious clay actually worked as a poison antidote. The dogs that were given the tablets survived their poisonings; the other dogs, well, not so much.

In the Renaissance, terra sigillata was used across Europe, not only as an antidote to poison, but also for the treatment of dysentery, ulceration, hemorrhages, gonorrhea, fever, kidney complaints, and eye infections. Most of these treatments would have been ineffective from a biological standpoint and were likely by-products of enthusiasm for these little clay tablets that sometimes worked as an antidote. If it's powerful enough to rescue someone poisoned by mercury sublimate, well, why not see if it works with gonorrhea as well?

After moving to the big leagues with his human trial in Hohenlohe, Berthold's fame and fortune grew. He became unstoppable as a one-man dirt-selling show in the late sixteenth century. Of course, an obvious problem with going into the clay-selling business is that it's not exactly a rare mineral. The stuff is pretty easy to find. So it was important for Berthold—and those who followed in his wake—to assign some special or, better yet,

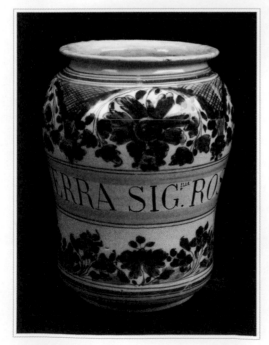

magical quality to their clay stores. Berthold claimed the special medicinal properties of his terra sigillata were owed to their geographic source in the hills around Striga.

In other words, this wasn't just any old dirt. You certainly weren't going to get the extraordinary medical benefits by digging in your neighbor's garden. No, you needed terra sigillata, the real stuff, specially stamped with a seal, drawn from the

Ceramic vase for terra sigillata storage.

THE DIRT-EATERS OF THE SOUTH

In 1984, the *New York Times* published an article on the declining trend of geophagy. If you think people would turn to eating a handful of soil in only the most dire circumstances, then you haven't met Mrs. Glass. "It just always tasted so good to me," said Mrs. Glass, a resident of rural Mississippi, in her interview with the *Times*. "When it's good and dug from the right place, dirt has a fine sour taste."

For many years, geophagy was part of the culinary tradition of the rural South, where the practice had been imported with the slave trade from West Africa. Dirt eating was relatively widespread in the late nineteenth and early twentieth centuries and almost exclusively engaged in by poor women who grew accustomed, even preferential, to the taste.

The same Mrs. Glass, who was at the time of her interview in the process of giving up the practice, wistfully added, "There are times when I really miss it. I wish I had some dirt right now."

The dirt of choice for Southerners was clay, which does in fact have some medicinal qualities to it; depending on the source, it can have high levels of calcium, copper, magnesium, iron, and zinc, all of which are important for human health, and, in the case of pregnant women—who occasionally engaged in geophagy across cultural groups—crucial for it. The soils of West Africa and the American South happen to be rich in these minerals, which might explain the development and continuation of the practice.

hills around Striga. Berthold's intelligent marketing plan was initially a success, and within a few years, Strigan terra sigillata was for sale at apothecary shops from Nuremberg to London.

The placebo effect was boosted by aesthetics: From Lemnos to Striga, the pieces of terra sigillata were also beautiful objects, so much so that part of their efficacy could be attributed to the patient's belief in a magical, almost talismanic quality of the little clay tablets.

There was even a special magic that resulted from just being near terra sigillata. Some physicians, hovering on the blurry renaissance line between science and magic, simply recommended that their patient wear a terra sigillata tablet around the neck to enjoy its curative properties.

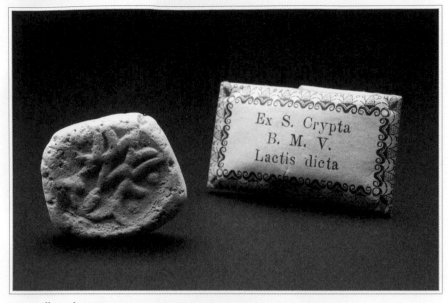

Terra sigillata, plus Latin.

It couldn't last forever, though, and soon many towns were getting in on the action, harvesting clay themselves, putting their own special stamp on it, and proclaiming their tablets held their own particular medicinal virtues. Berthold's empire began to crumble.

Poisoning gradually became less common (yay, humans!) and advances in medicine in the early modern era brought more effective treatments for dysentery, ulceration, hemorrhages, gonorrhea, fever, kidney complaints, and eye infections. And so terra sigillata gradually fell out of use, with the handful of tablets that survived getting picked up by wealthy antiquarians on Grand Tours of Europe in the nineteenth century and eventually making their way into curiosity cabinets and museums.

Eat Your Clay

Though unlikely to be recommended by your doctor, eating clay for medicinal purposes is still very much alive in alternative therapies. Proponents claim that ingesting clay can help your body detoxify by adsorbing, and then passing through, heavy metals that have accumulated in your insides.

The problem, however, is that we actually need some metals in our system — iron, for example — and clay is not very good at discriminating among metal types. It's also not always easy to know exactly what else is in the clay you're eating. It could carry parasites, bacteria, or even, ironically, heavy metals such as lead. As a result, the practice is not typically recommended by physicians today.

But that didn't stop actress Shailene Woodley from proclaiming her own experiments with clay eating in an interview on the *Late Show with David Letterman* and in a blog post for the beauty website *Into the Gloss* in 2014:

> So, I've discovered that clay is great for you because your body doesn't absorb it, and it apparently provides a negative charge, so it bonds to negative isotopes. And, this is crazy: It also helps clean heavy metals out of your body. My friend started eating it and the next day she called me and said, "Dude, my shit smells like metal." She was really worried, but we did some research together and everything said that when you first start eating clay, your bowel movements, pee, and even you, yourself, will smell like metal.

If you want to experiment with making your shit smell like metal, beware: Eating small amounts of processed clay is considered mostly harmless, but binge on the stuff and you'll end up with constipation . . . or worse. The best way to get calcium and other minerals is not from a pit you dig outside your house.

The Antidotes Hall of Shame

Poison is everywhere. Naturally or unnaturally, it can be in the soil (arsenic), in the air (carbon monoxide), in your drinks (lead), and in your food (cyanide). With so much danger around, it's no wonder humans have obsessed over finding a universal antidote—the one thing that could save us from all toxins. Imagine you're a medieval prince about to inherit the throne. Chances are, there are a lot of power-hungry wannabes waiting in the wings. A little arsenic or hemlock might be your best friend or your worst nightmare. Just in case, best have an antidote on standby.

For millennia, a certain amount of magical thinking was employed when arming oneself against poison because science was inconveniently slow to catch up. So grab your handy unicorn horn and a bezoar, and let's take a look.

BEZOARS

Bezoars have been used for centuries as antidotes to poisons. A bezoar is solid mass of undigested food, plant fibers, or hair found in the digestive tracts of animals, including deer, porcupines, fish, and, yes, humans. Anyone with a cat is familiar with the less-cool feline version: hairballs.

Bezoars and other stone-like items created by animals often had a good story behind them. Legends told of deer that would eat poisonous snakes and become immune or cry tears that solidified into poison-curing stones. First-century Arabic author al-Birumi claimed bezoars could protect against one poison called "the snot of Satan," which we hope *never ever* to encounter. By the

twelfth century, when Europe became plagued with, uh, plagues, the bezoar crept into pharmacopeias as panaceas and alexipharmics (poison antidotes).

Bezoars were a seductive notion for the rich and royal, who were at risk of assassination. The stones were often enclosed in bejeweled gold for display or worn as amulets. Indian bezoars, in particular, were sought for life-threatening fevers, poisonous bites, bleeding, jaundice, and melancholy. Consumers were also known to scrape off a bit of bezoar and add it to their drinks for heart health and kidney stones. These tonics were sometimes adulterated with toxic mercury or antimony, which caused vomiting and diarrhea, making buyers think they were effective.

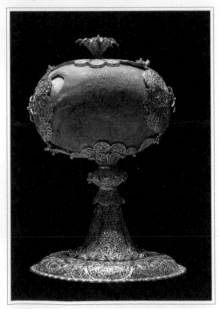

Indian bezoar mounted in gold, seventeenth century. Hairballs never looked so fancy.

But were they? One team of researchers soaked bezoars in an arsenic-laced solution and found that the stones absorbed the arsenic or that the poison was neutralized. Hard to say if it worked well enough to cure a fatal dose. Ambroise Paré, one of the preeminent French physicians of the sixteenth century, was also a doubter. The king's cook, who'd been stealing silver, was given the choice between hanging or being Paré's lab rat. He chose the latter. After the cook consumed poison, Paré looked on as a bezoar was stuffed down his throat. Six hours later, he died wracked with pain. Perhaps he chose . . . poorly?

MITHRIDATES

This antidote was named after Mithridates VI, the king of Pontus and Armenia Minor. Born in 134 BCE, he pretty much invented the phrase "what doesn't kill you makes you stronger" by consuming poisons daily to prevent his own assassination. His royal home was stocked with stingray spines, toxic mushrooms, scorpions, mineral poisons, and a poisonous plant–filled garden. He was so unpoisonable that after his son took over his kingdom and he faced execution, he couldn't even commit suicide by poison! He begged a guard to stab him to death. (It worked.)

Though the king's actual recipe for the antidote is nowhere to be found, versions began to circulate after his death, and they became synonymous with the king himself. Compounds with lengthy and expensive ingredient lists prevailed, including iris, cardamom, anise, frankincense, myrrh, ginger, and saffron. In the first century, Pliny the Elder snarkily remarked, "The Mithridatic antidote is composed of fifty-four ingredients. . . . Which of the gods, in the name of Truth, fixed these absurd proportions? . . . It is plainly a showy parade of the art, and a colossal boast of science."

Showy or not, people would take the extensive mix of herbs, pound them together with honey, and eat a nut-sized portion to cure themselves. At least it endowed them with expensive-smelling breath.

HORNS

Unicorn horns have been considered a part of antidote legend since the mythical beast galloped into literature around 300 BCE. For centuries afterward, real earthly beasts would sacrifice their lives and their horns to slake our thirst for the miraculous, nonexistent animal, including rhinoceroses, narwhals, and oryx. Even fossilized ammonites were used. It was believed that drinking vessels made of such horns might neutralize poisons, and wounds could be cured by holding them close by. In the sixteenth century, Mary, Queen of Scots reportedly used a unicorn horn to protect her from poisoning. Too bad it didn't prevent her beheading.

PEARLS

Pearls have long been thought to be powerful antidotes. A beautiful, rare gem created by the homely oyster, a pearl is born out of annoyance (the mollusk secretes iridescent nacre to cover an irritant, like a parasite or grain of sand). Pretty as they are, they're about as useful as the chalky antacid tablets on your bedside table; both are chiefly made of calcium carbonate. Good for a stomachache after some spicy food, but not exactly miraculous.

Pearl powder has been used in traditional Chinese medicine to treat a variety of diseases, and Ayurvedic physicians used it as an antidote in the

Middle Ages. It was also reported to make people immortal. An old Taoist recipe recommended taking a long pearl and soaking it in malt, "serpent's gall," honeycomb, and pumice stone. When softened, it would be pulled like taffy and cut into bite-sized pieces to eat, and voilà! You would suddenly no longer need food to stay alive. Cleopatra famously drank down a large and costly pearl dissolved in wine vinegar, though in that case she wasn't avoiding poison. She didn't want to lose a bet with Antony—which might have fatally injured her pride.

THERIAC

Theriac was an herbal concoction created in the first century by Emperor Nero's physician, Andromachus, who was reported to have Mithridates's secret notes. It was a mashed formula of about seventy ingredients, including cinnamon, opium, rose, iris, lavender, and acacia in a honey base. In the twelfth century, theriac made in Venice was branded as particularly special, and Venetian treacle (derived from a Middle English translation of *theriac*) became a hot commodity. Its public, dramatic production often attracted curious crowds.

By the eighteenth century, cheaper golden syrup was substituted for honey. As treacle began to lose its luster as a treatment, its definition as an herbal remedy disappeared from common vernacular. But the sweet syrup remained. Which is why when we think of treacle, we think of treacle tarts, not a fancy means of saving ourselves from a deathly poisoning.

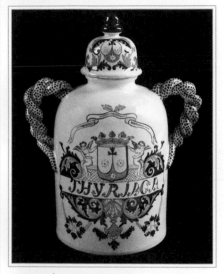

Tasty antidote, anyone?

WHAT ACTUALLY WORKS

Thankfully, science has brought us a wide range of antidotes for many items we shouldn't be exposed to in dangerous quantities, if at all. N-acetylcysteine, fondly referred to as NAC by doctors, saves us from acetaminophen overdoses. Ethanol can treat antifreeze poisoning. Atropine, ironically one of the main components of plants in the toxic nightshade family (such as mandrake), can treat poisoning from some dangerous fertilizers and chemical nerve agents used as weapons. For years, poisonings were treated with emetics, though it turns out that plain old carbon—in the form of activated charcoal—can adsorb poisons (the poisons stick to the surface of the charcoal) in the digestive system before they're dissolved and digested by the body.

As long as the natural world and its humans keep making things to kill us off, we'll keep developing methods to not die untimely deaths.

We'll just leave the fancy hairballs off the list.

Tools

Slicing, Dicing, Dousing, and Draining

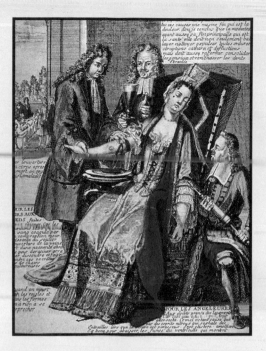

12

Bloodletting

Of Mozart's Requiem, Nonfunny Humors, the Origin of the Barber Pole, Real Iron Men, and George Washington's No Good, Very Bad Cold

In August 1791, at the age of thirty-five, an ailing Wolfgang Amadeus Mozart received a commission to compose a requiem mass for an anonymous patron. Mozart, who had been suffering from weight loss, anemia, headaches, and swoons, became paranoid that he was being commissioned to write his own requiem.

Weeks later, his already moody personality wasn't the only thing that worsened. By November, he was unable to leave his bed. Attacks of violent vomiting, diarrhea, and arthritis, plus swelling of his hands and feet, made it impossible to continue composing. The songs of his beloved pet canary became insufferable. He was convinced he was being poisoned.

His physicians tried to save him, but one of the popular treatments at the time may have been the very cause of his demise: bloodletting. Some have estimated that he may have

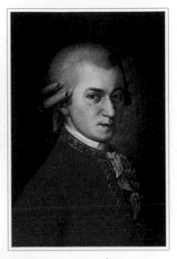

A posthumous portrait of Mozart.

lost more than four pints of blood in his last week of life. His sister-in-law, Sophie Haibel, noted, "They bled him and applied cold compresses to his head, whereupon his forces visibly forsook him and he lost consciousness, which he never recovered." Mozart died twenty-four hours later and was buried in an unmarked grave.

Without an autopsy, no one will ever know the true cause of his death, but many believe with certainty that bloodletting helped end an extraordinary life.

BAD BLOOD

Blood leaking out of the lanced arms of sick patients. The smell of iron in the air. The sticky drip of liquid into a ceramic collecting bowl, notched on the sides to fit a limp arm. Today, the act of cutting into a blood vessel to spill blood—*on purpose, voluntarily*—is worth a modern head-shake of incredulity. Since antiquity, blood has been considered the essential component of life. Even the Bible states that "the life of flesh is in the blood," which makes the practice of bloodletting so fascinating. After all, why on earth remove what you need to live?

First, you have to put yourself in the mindset of ancient physicians. The earliest evidence of bloodletting—among Egyptians around 1500 BCE—is from a time when the inner workings of the body were a mystery. They were drawing conclusions from limited information. Ancient Romans had thought that a woman's menses was a natural way to remove toxins from the body, so removing blood from people seemed a reasonable way to keep one healthy. And because this was long before we discovered that blood *circulates* throughout the body, texts from the Han Dynasty (206 BCE–220 CE) discuss how blood could become "stagnant" and how removing old, "decayed" blood was one way to fix this stasis.

Or maybe the sick were just imbalanced and in need of a good purge. So went the theories of Hippocrates and his four humors. Too much blood, phlegm, yellow bile, or black bile? Purge via bleeding, vomiting, or clearing the bowels.

Also a fan of the whole "too much blood" theory, Erasistratus—who didn't even advocate bloodletting—inadvertently gave the practice a boost in the third century BCE by proposing that many illnesses stemmed from *plethora*, or being overloaded with blood. Although he recommended vomiting, diet, or exercise to fix plethora, many physicians turned to bloodletting.

It was only a matter of time before we entered cure-all territory. In the second century CE, Galen declared that bleeding was the solution for everything wrong with the body—including *hemorrhage*. Let that one stew for a while.

Anatomy and physiology had a ways to go, obviously.

Often, bloodletting was done in a reasonable fashion—excluding young children and the very old or trying to avoid removing excessive amounts—but that wasn't always the case. There were plenty of gory missteps on our way to modern phlebotomy. Sure, the *why* behind bloodletting was disturbing, but the *how* was pretty skin-crawling, too.

So, who was doing all this bleeding anyway?

TOOLS OF A BLOOD-SOAKED TRADE

Anything that could cut was used for bloodletting. Animal teeth, stones, sharpened pieces of wood, quills, shells. As the process evolved, so did the tools. By the seventeenth century, practitioners had the procedure down to a science: First, a tourniquet would be applied, then the upper arm's basilic vein would be slit open. And what was used to slice into that vein? Let's see. . . .

The **lancet** was one of the more sophisticated tools of the last few centuries. It was a curved or pointed blade on the end of a handle. To this day, one of the most popular international medical journals is named after this beloved instrument: *The Lancet*. Thumb lancets were pocket-sized versions that folded into a pretty ivory or tortoiseshell case for the fashionable bleeder on the go.

The **fleam** was a multi-bladed, multi-sized contraption used for larger cuts and often for bleeding larger subjects like horses.

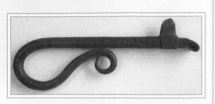

A *thirteenth-century iron fleam.*

With a name that could be mistaken for a 1980s horror movie, the **scarificator** was a box with multiple spring-loaded blades, often used prior to cupping (inducing a vacuum under a glass cup) in order to draw more blood.

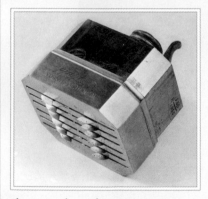

The *exterior of a scarificator.*

Every tool had its loyal fans. J. E. Snodgrass proclaimed in 1841 his adoration for his spring-loaded lancet:

> I love thee, bloodstain'd, faithful friend! . . .
> And I shall love thee to the Last!

Perhaps there was no one at the time to tell him *Get thee a room.*

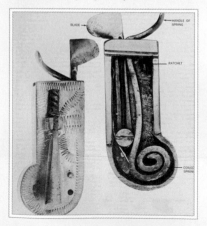

A *spring-loaded lancet.*

SHAVE AND A HAIRCUT AND A BLEEDING

In ancient Rome, multitalented stylists known as *tonsures* were responsible for polishing up their clients by cutting hair, trimming nails and calluses, yanking bad teeth, and bloodletting. For a price, you came away with a mani-pedi, a gap-toothed grin, and a case of anemia.

In medieval Europe, the barber-surgeon became the go-to person for not only cosmetic services, but amputations, cupping, leeching, and boil drain

ing. Smallpox a problem? Bleed it away. Epilepsy? Bleed that, too. Plague? Step on in, ignore the bloody rags on the floor, and please don't die in my chair.

Initially, the shedding of blood was often done by the clergy for themselves and others. Monks and clerics were celibate, and bloodletting seemed to tame their libidos further (the anti-Viagra of the day!). But after 1163, Pope Alexander III forbade the clergy from involving themselves in studies of a physical nature. The canon declared that "the church abhors blood" and thereafter clerics did not perform surgery or bloodletting, nor did they study anatomy. In England, barber-surgeons took up the role. The bloodletter would

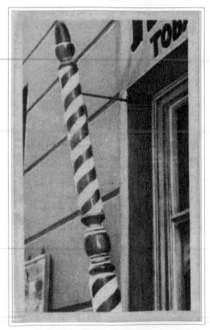

The classic barber pole, a vestige of the profession's role in bloodletting.

smell, touch, and taste the blood (let's heave a collective *ewww* here) to diagnose the patient. Bowls of blood would sit on barbers' windowsills to attract customers before a law was passed that required them to quietly pitch the blood into the River Thames instead.

The modern barber pole, already becoming an antique in our day with its twirling red, blue, and white (or just red and white), is a throwback to these barber-surgeons, who placed the poles outside their place of work to advertise their vocation. The pole symbolized the stick that a patient would squeeze to facilitate the bleeding process, with a bowl at the bottom to catch the spilled liquid. Some say the white stripe symbolized the tourniquet, the blue represented the vein, and the red, blood.

Next time you go to your barber, maybe ask for a good bleeding and see if he gets the historical joke.

BLEED YOURSELF TO BLISS

It's the seventeenth century and you've been dumped by the gent you thought was surely The One. Oh, what could fix this broken heart? Some brandy and gossip with a good friend? A pint of the Baroque-era equivalent of Ben & Jerry's? Close! A broken heart does call for a pint of something; it's just not as pleasant as Chunky Monkey.

In 1623, French physician Jacques Ferrand wrote an entire book on surgical cures for lovesickness, particularly if the sufferer was "plump and well fed." He recommended bloodletting to the point of heart failure (literal heart failure, that is) and noted that "the opening of the hemorrhoids is the surest remedy." Because somehow he had figured out that heartbreak and hemorrhoids go hand in hand.

This wasn't the first time bloodletting entered the realm of mental health. Like anatomy, psychology had also long been a mystery to doctors. Confusing and seemingly incurable ailments like heartbreak, melancholy, and mania had many a physician reaching for his lancet. The *Huang Di Nei Jing* texts from the Han Dynasty prescribed bloodletting for symptoms of "incessant laughing" or mania, because a little hemorrhage was sure to quiet you down. Later, Galen had thought that different types of "insanity"—frenzy, mania, melancholy, and fatuity (foolishness)—were due to humoral imbalances and, thus, they required bleeding.

In the eighteenth century, one of the most infamous psychiatric hospitals in the world, St. Mary of Bethlehem in London, was notoriously nicknamed "Bedlam" for the horrific behaviors, conditions, and treatments found within. Writer Alexander Cruden was institutionalized multiple times for shocking behaviors such as attempting to date widows and getting upset over incest. How dare he? He had noted that "The common Prescriptions of a Bethlemitical Doctor are a Purge and a Vomit, and a Vomit and a Purge over again, and sometimes a Bleeding." This was sadly before aerosolized room deodorizer was invented.

Benjamin Rush, physician and founding father, recommended "heroic depletion therapy" (see Mercury, page 3) for many ailments, including this prescription for mania: "20 to 40 ounces of blood [two and a half pints] may be taken at once . . . early and copious bleeding are wonderful in calming people." He's sort of correct. After all, people of all temperaments are calm when they're too fatigued and anemic to care.

Even the *Sushruta Samhita*, the ancient Sanskrit text, remarked that bloodletting is followed by a sense of cheerfulness upon the patient. And who doesn't want that? Pass the knife.

Well, maybe not just yet. Here are a few people who probably wouldn't describe their experience as "cheery."

THE EXSANGUINATED LIVES OF THE RICH AND FAMOUS

Marie Antoinette was bled after she gave birth before a room full of courtly observers. (If you think this is impressive, remember that if she'd had social media, she could've given birth in front of *millions*.) The queen ended up fainting and was revived by bloodletting, or at least the pain of it.

Some had far worse outcomes, especially when bloodletting was employed as a desperate last resort. In 1685, Charles II of England succumbed to "fits" while shaving. His fourteen physicians were under great pressure to keep him alive. Besides bleeding, the poor king endured enemas, purgatives, and cupping, and had to eat the gallstone of an East Indian goat. Plasters made from pigeon droppings were thoughtfully applied to his feet. They bled copious amounts from him again and again, once even slitting open his jugular veins. At the end, he was left nearly bloodless before he died, though perhaps his soul was simply running screaming from the bird-poop poultices. Thirty years later, Charles II's niece, Queen Anne—then on the throne herself—was bled and purged after having fits and falling unconscious; she survived only two days after the doctors arrived.

Lord Byron, suffering from a violent cold complete with fevers and body aches, had an ongoing battle with his physicians about bloodletting. He adamantly refused, stating that it hadn't helped in previous illnesses. Finally, he gave in to their nagging and proclaimed, "Come as you are; I see a damned set

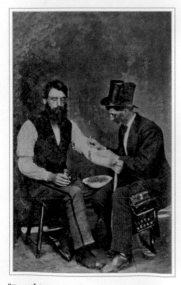

"*Breathing a vein*" in 1860.

of butchers. Take away as much blood as you will but have done with it." After several pints were bled over the course of three bleedings, his physicians were surprised that Byron worsened. Desperate, the doctors blistered him and applied leeches around his ears. Lord Byron died soon after, and his physicians promptly blamed him for putting off the bleeding for too long.

George Washington was yet another famous victim of bloodletting. Three years after retiring from his presidency, he came down with a fever after riding in snowy weather. He had trouble breathing, probably

AN ARRAY OF
BLOODLETTING INSTRUMENTS

PHLEBOTOMY

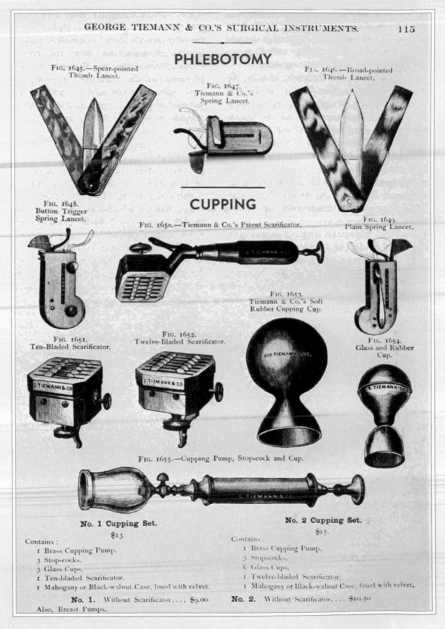

FIG. 1645.—Spear-pointed Thumb Lancet.

FIG. 1647. Tiemann & Co.'s Spring Lancet.

FIG. 1646.—Broad-pointed Thumb Lancet.

FIG. 1648. Button Trigger Spring Lancet.

CUPPING

FIG. 1650.—Tiemann & Co.'s Patent Scarificator.

FIG. 1649. Plain Spring Lancet.

FIG. 1653. Tiemann & Co.'s Soft Rubber Cupping Cup.

FIG. 1651. Ten-Bladed Scarificator.

FIG. 1652. Twelve-Bladed Scarificator.

FIG. 1654. Glass and Rubber Cup.

FIG. 1655.—Cupping Pump, Stop-cock and Cup.

No. 1 Cupping Set.
$13.

Contains:
1 Brass Cupping Pump.
3 Stop-cocks.
3 Glass Cups.
1 Ten-bladed Scarificator.
1 Mahogany or Black-walnut Case, lined with velvet.

No. 1. Without Scarificator.... $9.00

Also, Breast Pumps.

No. 2 Cupping Set.
$15.

Contains:
1 Brass Cupping Pump.
3 Stop-cocks.
6 Glass Cups.
1 Twelve-bladed Scarificator.
1 Mahogany or Black-walnut Case, lined with velvet.

No. 2. Without Scarificator.... $10.50

from a bout of severe epiglottitis. His physicians aggressively bled him, tried a drink of molasses, vinegar, and butter (which nearly choked him to death), blistered him, bled him again, tried laxatives and emetics, and bled him some more for good measure. A day later, he was bled yet again. All told, he may have been bled of five to nine pints of blood and died shortly after. Quite a price to pay for an illness that started out as a bad cold.

The Bleeding Slows to a Trickle

Even in the face of his critics, Dr. Benjamin Rush maintained his staunch and loud defense of bloodletting, and his landscaping proved this. At the height of the Yellow Fever epidemic in Philadelphia, his front lawn had so much congealed, spilled blood that it stank and buzzed with flies. No show on HGTV could have fixed that disaster. Unfortunately for Rush's patients, the doctor greatly overestimated the body's blood volume—by 200 percent. He would often remove four to six pints of blood in a single day (the average human male has about twelve pints). And remember, he'd often bleed several days in a row. His treatment mortality rate was so high that a critic named William Cobbett decried, "The times are ominous indeed, when quack to quack cries purge and bleed." Cobbett even went so far as to say that Rush's so-called heroic therapy was "a perversion of nature's healing powers." *Burn!*

Though bleeding was a well-loved weapon among physicians for more than two millennia, detractors like Cobbett were always around. Erasistratus thought blood loss would weaken patients (he was right). In the seventeenth century, an Italian scholar named Ramazzini claimed, "It seems as if the phlebotomist [blood-letter] grasped the Delphic Sword in his hand to exterminate the innocent."

By the eighteenth and nineteenth centuries, opposition from many physicians and scientists began to turn the tide of change. Louis Pasteur and Robert Koch showed that inflammation came from infection and wouldn't be cured with bloodletting. In 1855, John Hughes Bennett, a physician from

Edinburgh, used statistics to show that pneumonia mortality decreased as bloodletting declined. With the current understanding of human physiology and pathology, medical practices in the West began to move away from the antiquated ideas of humoral medicine.

Today, bloodletting, or *phlebotomy* as it's called (Greek for "cutting a blood vessel"), is still used throughout the world. California had to ban bloodletting by acupuncturists in 2010. And it's still a modern practice with Unani, a Persian-Arabic branch of medicine that traces its roots back to the thirteenth century. Bleeding with suction cup therapy, *wet-cupping*, is also still done in traditional Arabic medicine, with some positive studies. (In the 2016 Summer Olympics, swimmer Michael Phelps was seen covered with bruises from "dry cupping," using just suction without the bleeding.)

With our modern understanding of the human body, it would make sense that bloodletting might improve symptoms of high blood pressure and occasionally heart failure; instead, we have non-invasive pills that don't require slitting a vein wide open. But for some diseases, bloodletting remains a suitable remedy. Hemochromatosis, a disorder that causes dangerous over-accumulation of iron, is treated with regular bleeding that depletes the body of this element. Phlebotomy can also be used for polycythemia vera, which causes a pathologic increase in red blood cells. After all Galen wrote, it turns out that too much blood is truly a bloody problem to have.

Pity that the bloodletters of the past didn't realize that most of the time, blood is best left *inside* the body, rather than outside.

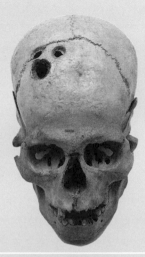

13

Lobotomy

Of Ancient Holey Heads,
the Stone of Madness, Neural Eggbeaters,
Kitchen Ice Picks, and Walter Freeman's Lobotomobile

No one doubts that the Kennedys were America's own royal family. Handsome and beautiful, well bred and well connected, they had the money, pedigree, smarts, and political ties to leave an indelible mark on our nation's history and cultural consciousness. They also had secrets to hide.

For decades, Rosemary Kennedy was the least known of all the siblings of John F. Kennedy. Photos of her appearance at King George and Queen Elizabeth's court in 1938 show her smiling, her dark hair coiffed perfectly, white gloves and couture gown fitting her curvy frame to perfection. The British press was wild for her beauty. Eligible young men wooed her at events. At first glance, she easily outshone her own patrician mother and plainer sister, Kathleen.

But what most didn't know is that much of Rosemary's inner world was kept a secret. Her birth had been delayed and her mother held her legs closed until the doctor could arrive two hours later—on the advisement of a nurse and despite the fact that the baby was crowning. Many blame this for Rose's mental deficiencies, perhaps from lack of oxygen during those crucial hours. Her siblings were athletes and achievers, but Rosemary didn't hit her developmental milestones on time, if at all. As an adult, she possessed the intelligence of a fourth grader and wrote letters with simplistic handwriting riddled with spelling errors. Her father, Joe Kennedy, ambassador to England, can be seen grasping her arm tightly in a few photographs, evidence of his attempts to keep Rosemary's behavior in check.

By her early twenties, all the cognitive gains from years of tutoring and constant vigilance were slowly slipping away. She'd escape her convent boarding school and wander the streets at night. Her unexpected outbursts of emotion—sometimes yelling, sometimes punching (and the punches hurt, for she was strong and healthy)—were becoming too difficult to contain. For an elite Boston family as socially active as the Kennedys were, having an uncontrollable child with "disgraceful" mental deficiencies could amount to social suicide. They just needed her to be calm, predictable, and more . . . Kennedy-like.

It just so happened that a new neurosurgical technique was stirring up excitement and interest. A *Saturday Evening Post* article in 1941 claimed that it could help patients who were "problems to their families and nuisances to themselves."

Joe Kennedy called Dr. Walter Freeman for help, unbeknownst to his wife, who was overseas. In November 1941, Rosemary Kennedy was lobotomized, and she disappeared from the public eye.

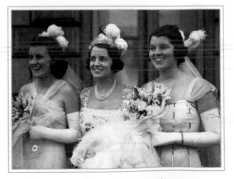

Kathleen, Rose, and Rosemary Kennedy in 1938.

A BRIEF HISTORY OF HOLEY HEADS

The oldest form of surgery, trepanning (also called trephining, both from the Greek word *trypanon*, meaning to drill or bore) was performed by scraping the skull away, cutting a square shape to remove the center, drilling a circlet of tiny holes like stamp perforations, or drilling out a circle. The tools used could be flint, obsidian, metal, or shell. Supposedly, this wasn't brain surgery. No joke intended—really, it wasn't. The brain, its blood vessels, and the skinlike covering, the meninges, weren't touched. People seemed to understand that if you stirred up some brain pudding, bad things happened.

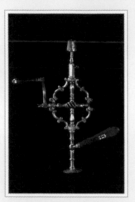

Why was the procedure done? For a lot of good reasons: There is plenty of evidence that they were performed after skull fractures, possibly to remove broken fragments and alleviate pressure by removing blood clots. In fact, plenty of skulls showed evidence of healing bone, which means the patients survived.

The bad reasons for trepanning? Random headaches. Epilepsy. Melancholy. Mental illness. And also—minor head injuries. Hippocrates recommended the procedure when all that was suffered was a bump on the head. Just in case. (Suddenly, the quip "I need that like I need a hole in the head" makes a little more sense.)

During the Renaissance, the use of firearms increased the number of traumatic head injuries and treatment with trepanning. Unfortunately, by the eighteenth century, trepanning had become a dangerous prospect. Pre-antisepsis Europe was a rather dirty place. Some estimated that 50 percent of those trepanned died (unlike the ancient skulls found before—which boasted closer to a 20 percent mortality rate). It was such a barbaric situation that in 1839, surgeon Sir Astley Cooper argued, "If you were to trephine, you ought to be trephined in turn."

Though trepanning is still used for treatment of traumatic brain injury, an occasional few have veered from this obvious lifesaving strategy and instead bored themselves for a buzz. In 1965, a Dutchman named Bart Huges thought it could bring him to a higher state of consciousness. Using an electric drill, knife, and hypodermic needle, he went to work. Afterward, he stated, "I feel as I felt before the age of fourteen." (As if we wanted to relive our most awkward hormonal teen years—*forever*.) This incident occurred after he failed out of medical school and before he went on to write *Trepanation: The Cure for Psychosis*. Others followed suit, but luckily most reasonable people prefer LSD to neurosurgery for existential psychedelic assistance. It's much less messy.

DRILLING TO THE ROOT OF MADNESS

To better understand Rosemary's fate, we need to crank back the timeline to the origins of brain surgery, the first kind of surgery ever, actually: the practice of trepanning (see box "A Brief History of Holey Heads," opposite). Trepanning is the process of creating a hole in the skull. It's the earliest recorded surgical procedure in history. Skulls from Mesolithic times (possibly as far back as 0000 to 10,000 BCE) unequivocally show signs of the procedure, which we know was practiced in several ancient civilizations, including Mesoamerica, Greece, the Roman Empire, India, and China.

For every sound use of trepanning, such as removing pieces of bone in skull fractures or relieving pressure, there were plenty of misfires. The good news was that people rightly theorized that the brain was the seat of thought and emotion; the bad news was that we had horrific methods of fixing a disordered thought process. A twelfth-century Greek surgeon recommended trepanning for melancholy and madness. A thirteenth-century Greek surgical text recommended that those with epilepsy be trepanned so that "the humors and air may go out and evaporate." As easy as letting the air out of a balloon, right? Demons causing sickness were also thought to skeddadle with a little help from a cranial escape hatch.

During the Renaissance, a theory emerged that a stone residing within the brain was the seat of madness, idiocy, and dementia. Remove it and you might prevent the befouling of the rest of the mind. In Hieronymus Bosch's 1475 painting *Cutting the Stone*, also called *The Extraction of the Stone of Madness*, a poor soul sits tied to a fancy chair, gazing with a decided side-eye at the viewer. A doctor (who, for unknown reasons, is wearing a metal funnel) is cutting into his head. Multiple other works of art during this and the next century depict this hopeful surgery. It's unclear if the paintings were theatrical in nature or depicted true surgical attempts at removing that dratted (and nonexistent) rock.

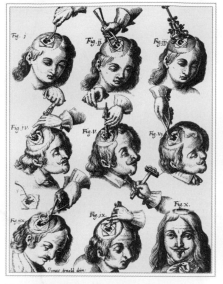

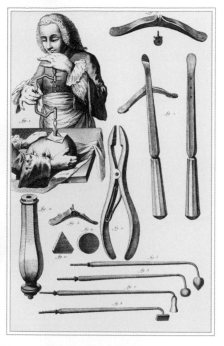

Trepanning demo and tools, for the DIYer.

Life came to imitate art, however, when Swiss doctor Gottlieb Burckhardt sliced into six brains in 1888. With no surgical experience, Burckhardt operated on patients with schizophrenia and psychotic hallucinations. Like the ancient doctors of yore, he used a trephine (basically, a round cookie-cutter-like bone saw on a stick) to drill holes near the temples, but here's where he departed: He then cut through the brain's dura and scooped out parts of the cerebral cortex with, in some cases, a sharp spoon. Yes, *spoonfuls of brain were removed*. Though some of the patients became "quieter" and no longer hallucinated, many were left with lingering neurological problems, died from ensuing complications, or even committed suicide. A psychiatrist at the time commented that "[Burckhardt] suggested that restless patients could be pacified by scratching away the cerebral cortex."

Burckhardt's procedure was the first lobotomy, though that term wouldn't be coined until decades later. Unlike trepanning, which aimed only at opening a hole in the skull without disturbing the brain or its meningeal covering, this new approach to surgery was a whole other kettle of, er, spoons. (And ice picks. And egg beaters. More on these other tools shortly.) It also marked the dawn of psychosurgery—damaging the brain on purpose to cure mental illness—a new invention that accompanied exciting discoveries about the links between our brains and behaviors (see box "Phineas Gage, the Hot Dude with a Hole in His Head," page 147), and other developments in neuroanatomy.

The medical community thought Burckhardt barbaric and received his work with cold horror. He never performed the procedures again. It would be almost fifty years before someone tried another lobotomy.

What changed? The world had entered a mental health crisis.

THE LOBOTOMY: AN AMERICAN (STOLEN) INVENTION

In the later 1930s and early 1940s, physicians in the United States were desperate. The number of institutionalized mentally ill patients grew to more than four hundred thousand. Psychiatric patients took up more than half of the hospital beds across the country. There were no good pharmacological treatments, and these patients took enormous emotional, physical, and financial tolls on families and the asylums. Patients were treated in often horrific conditions. Their savior? A gout-ridden Portuguese neuroscientist with a syringe full of booze.

In 1935, Egas Moniz attempted another psychosurgical cure for mental illness. the leucotomy (Greek for "cutting the white," as in the white matter of the brain). The first patient chosen was an institutionalized woman suffering from years of debilitating depression. His own hands deformed by gout, Moniz employed a surgeon to drill a hole in the patient's brain near the top of the head and inject pure ethanol to kill parts of the frontal lobe. (Yes, it's the same alcohol found in your wine, but no, you won't kill your brain cells after a glassful of rosé. So stop panicking.)

In later procedures, they used an instrument called a leucotome, which was a nifty metal rod that, when pushed into your squishy brain, would shoot out a wire loop that spun around and got a nice churn going. It was less like an eggbeater scrambling a good flan, and more like a melon baller used on an overripe cantaloupe. The brain texture was later described by American surgeon James Watts as "what butter's like when it's been out of the refrigerator for a while." There you go. Now we've ruined flan, cantaloupe, and butter, too.

Moniz was later given the Nobel Prize for his work, despite the fact that many of his patients ended up right back at the asylums where they started. Although the medical community was yet again horrified, Moniz did not back away like Burckhardt. He spread the word.

One of the doctors who listened to Moniz's gospel was Walter Freeman, the American neurologist who would eventually lobotomize Rosemary Kennedy. Freeman partnered with neurosurgeon James Watts to continue Moniz's work on American soil. In 1936, after their first patient survived and seemed cured (her anxiety diminished, and she seemed healthy but "shrewish and demanding with her husband"), they moved onward. But many patients had zero or only fleeting improvement. Many lost spontaneity. Hallucinations often continued.

These setbacks didn't stop the optimistic duo. After only six operations, Freeman and Watts went on an aggressive publicity campaign to show what they'd done. Articles popped up in the *Washington Post* and *Time* magazine. "Doctors with pocketbooks filled and minds agog" were reported to have attended meetings in droves. No matter that they'd had a terrible setback with their fifth patient, who showed no improvement but *gained* epilepsy and incontinence.

They soon became celebrities, and Freeman even coined a new term for the surgery: *lobotomy*. By rebranding Moniz's leucotomy, Freeman distanced himself from the Portuguese doctor, and in doing so, the term became closely associated with him. Well played, Dr. Freeman. He was a brilliant publicist

PHINEAS GAGE, THE HOT DUDE WITH A HOLE IN HIS HEAD

On September 13, 1848, a handsome foreman named Phineas Gage was working for a railroad company in Vermont. He and his team would drill holes into bedrock, lower in explosives, fill the hole with sand, and tamp it all down with an iron rod.

That was how it was supposed to work. Gage was lightly tamping down the powder before adding the sand, and in a moment of distraction, he turned his head to check on his men, skull poised above the javelin-like iron rod. As the rod accidentally scraped the side of the hole, it sparked against the rock, and the ensuing explosion sent the rod blasting through his left cheek, behind his left eye, and through the top of his head.

Miraculously, he woke up moments later. After a few convulsions, he was able to speak. His left eyeball protruded out of the socket. Brain tissue was smeared along the rod, which had landed eighty feet away. The town doctor examined him soon after and noted that "Mr. G got up and vomited. The effort of vomiting pressed out about half a teacupful of the brain, which fell upon the floor." Splat.

What was most interesting, aside from his survival, was the change in his personality. Before the accident, he possessed "a well-balanced mind . . . shrewd, smart . . . very energetic." Afterward, he became "fitful, irreverent, indulging at times in the grossest profanity (which was not previously his custom), manifesting but little deference for his fellows, impatient of restraint or

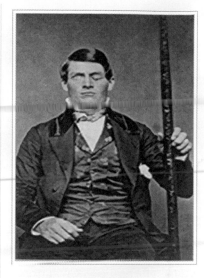

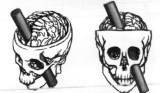

The path of the tamping iron through Gage's skull.

advice. . . . A child in his intellectual capacity and manifestations, he has the animal passions of a strong man."

Gage, as they said, "was no longer Gage." He would become a fascinating case study in the understanding of brain physiology and set the stage for more scientific exploration of frontal lobe surgery.

and salesman as well, sending out thousands of letters and articles to psychiatric institutions across the United States and taking every opportunity to speak out about the procedure.

In 1938, Freeman and Watts decided to change the surgery. Instead of burr holes at the top of the skull, they began to operate at the temples. Moniz's leucotome was not rigid enough for the procedure. Sometimes, it broke off in the brain. Instead, they used what looked like a narrow butter knife. This was the exact instrument used on Rosemary Kennedy. According to Kate Clifford Larsen's biography of Rosemary, the "quarter-inch-wide flexible spatula" was inserted through the burr holes in her temples. "Watts turned and scraped as he moved deeper into her brain." Rosemary was told to recite stories, verses, and even sing a song during the procedure. But after one slice too many, "she became incoherent. She slowly stopped talking."

Rosemary, as they knew her, was gone.

She couldn't walk or speak after the surgery and was institutionalized forever after. She disappeared from the Kennedy family's letters, as if forcibly forgotten. But these "setbacks" didn't stop Freeman. He was about to embark on some major updates to the procedure.

FREEMAN GOES SOLO

One day Freeman was going through his kitchen drawer and found an ice pick. It was the perfect instrument, he thought. Sharp, but not too sharp; strong, with just the right girth. Moniz's leucotome had a habit of breaking, and the butter knife method required the pesky addition of an actual *neurosurgeon*. Freeman decided he didn't need those complications.

And thus began the "ice-pick lobotomy."

After rendering his patients unconscious with electroshock therapy, Freeman would access the frontal lobes by lifting the eyelid, inserting the ice pick, tapping it gently with a hammer to poke through the thin orbital bone

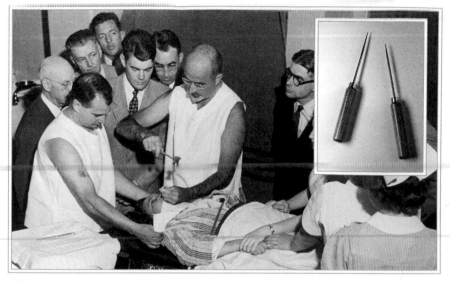

Walter Freeman performing a lobotomy. Inset: His trusty ice picks.

above the eyeball, and impaling the brain tissue (here, he usually paused to snap a photograph). He'd swish the ice pick left, right, up, down, and then repeat the procedure on the other side. The patient would leave with raccoon-bruised eyes and hopefully a calmer demeanor.

His former partner, Watts, was furious that this new approach didn't require an operating room or him, but Freeman didn't care. He was now free to do as many lobotomies as he could, while touting his miracle treatment around the country. He even had a car he called the "lobotomobile," which he had outfitted with all of his equipment to use as he traveled. He referred to his lobotomized patients as "trophies." Oh, the hubris!

Freeman wasn't without opponents, though. Many thought that slicing and scrambling brain tissue could not, by definition, bring back normalcy. Doctors verbally attacked him at American Medical Association (AMA) meetings. One physician later lamented, "It does disturb me to see the number of zombies that these operations turn out. I would guess that lobotomies going on all over the world have caused more mental invalids than they've cured."

Although his methods were callous, Freeman was no charlatan. He truly believed the lobotomy would solve psychiatry's biggest impediment—the sheer number of sick patients burdening families and societies. But more than a few patients became completely incapacitated by the procedure or died from hemorrhage. An undue proportion of patients were female. Even children, whose brains were not completely developed, were lobotomized, the youngest a mere four years old. "Troublesome" relatives or children with low IQs or difficult temperaments were lobotomized, like poor Rosemary Kennedy. Howard Dully, who wrote an autobiography entitled *My Lobotomy*, was a mentally sound twelve-year-old whose stepmother despised him and his imperfect behavior. She wanted a lobotomy performed on him despite six psychiatrists stating that Howard had no mental illness. Four told her that *she* was the one needing treatment. She convinced Freeman to perform the lobotomy, anyway.

And you thought evil stepmothers were only in fairy tales.

Psychosurgery Today

Freeman continued to perform lobotomies until his last procedure killed a woman in 1967 from cerebral hemorrhage. But the use of the lobotomy procedure had already been dying a slow death. Why? Because of the birth of a little pill called chlorpromazine, trade name Thorazine (named after the Norse god of thunder, Thor). Thorazine was the first effective antipsychotic, and though it wasn't perfect, it was far more humane than the lobotomy.

Neurosurgery today is a finely tuned, intimidating, and exacting science, far removed from the skull-scraping procedures of the past. As for psychosurgery? Today's better understanding of the complexities of the brain, mental illness, and the arsenal of multidisciplinary therapists and medications have transformed psychiatry. Surgical procedures do exist, but their use is scant.

The ice picks, thankfully, are long gone.

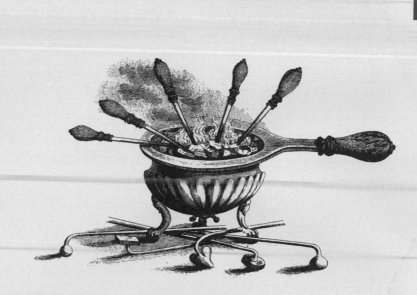

14

Cautery & Blistering

Of Hot Heads, Boiling Oil, Rude Coma Awakenings, Spanish Fly, and Flossing Peas through Your Pus

Let's say you have a nagging headache. Which would you prefer?

1. A glowing, red-hot iron applied to your temple until it chars your skin
2. Boiling oil dripped onto your forehead, making your epidermis die and peel off
3. Glittering green beetle paste gooped onto your scalp until it blisters and oozes
4. Some ibuprofen, a nap in a quiet room, and world peace

If you picked 4, then you clearly are missing out on some horrific remedies. The very idea of using these treatments is puzzling. When it comes to blistering, most people want to keep their skin intact, preferably not bubbling full of pus or watery ooze. And cautery? Well, one of the main jobs of the human nervous system is to jerk your hand away from that burning hot pot handle you just touched. Aerobic exercise aside, no one truly wants to feel the burn. But these "cures" were commonly used to treat every human condition, from fatigue to lovesickness. Ready for some sizzling flesh and blister popping? Read on, friend.

Ye Olde Arte of Making Yew Screame

Using burning-hot metal or electrically induced cautery to stop bleeding, slice through flesh, char a tumor to death, or annihilate whatever is making a wound fester—these all make scientific sense. In fact, cautery is commonly and successfully used in surgery today for many of these reasons. For the last few millennia, however, it wasn't so neat a procedure. Even when physicians' intentions were good, their tools were just too crude to execute the task in a way that was anything other than nightmarish. How nightmarish? Let's take a quick look at the history of burning humans.

When searing flesh physically with hot metal or electricity, the procedure is termed *actual cautery*. If you're imagining your favorite cooking show where you're told to "sear the meat to seal in the juices," well, you're not far off. Just replace "meat" with "human" and "seal in the juices" with "burn the hell out of whatever is bothering them." Delicious!

How was it done? Let's say you're a scullery maid with a pounding headache and you chose option 1 earlier. The physician or apothecary would shove a long iron rod (or, less commonly, copper or platinum if he was feeling fancy) into the fireplace or a hot coal–filled brazier. When the instrument was heated to red-hot, he'd lay it on your temple until it sizzled and

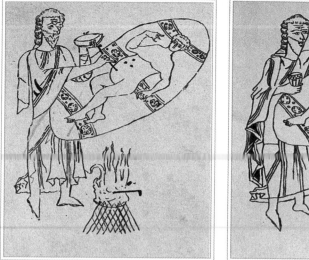

Tenth-century depiction of cautery on a surfboard. JK.

fried the skin. And if you had an open wound on your noggin? The doctor would burn the open ends of blood vessels to closure, vaporizing the wound to dryness, and if all went well, leaving a good smoky char behind. You'd be screaming bloody murder, but hey, at least you're alive! (For now.) As for the headache, who the hell cares? You're too busy dealing with that charred skin on your face.

Or perhaps you picked option 2? You're the lucky winner of the *potential cautery* package! This technique involves burning flesh chemically with "gentler" methods such as acids and boiling oil. First, you would lie down while your physician heated the oil in a copper flask. Once it was boiling—think french fry–friendly temperatures—he'd pour a tiny amount into a smaller vessel and then drip-drip-drip it onto your forehead. And if the situation called for a caustic substance, he'd place a tiny nugget of a burning chemical beneath a bandaged plaster. Unlike actual cautery, this would be a far slower flavor of torture because it took time for the caustic to dissolve and burn the tissue.

Obviously, both types of cautery didn't always go as planned. If the charred flesh stuck to the iron, the wound would be torn wide open when the iron was removed. Too bad nonstick cooking spray was unavailable then. You were left bleeding and with an even larger wound—not exactly the point of cauterizing to begin with. And if the iron wasn't heated to the right temperature, the whole process "begets nothing but pain and anguish," claimed seventeenth-century surgeon James Yonge. If that wasn't enough, there could be fevers, terrible scars, and death after cautery was applied. It also didn't always fix the problem. When using boiling oil, the oil might drip onto perfectly normal tissue, causing "pains, inflammations, and other horride symptomes," according to famed French surgeon Ambroise Paré.

Did we mention that there was a lot of screaming involved?

FIRE CURES AND
OTHER PAINFUL PRESCRIPTIONS

You might be wondering what kind of monster would subject his patients to such pain. The founding father of medicine, for one. In the fourth century BCE, Hippocrates used red-hot irons to incinerate painful hemorrhoids (or piles, as hemorrhoids were once called). "When the cautery is applied," he directed, "the patient's head and hands should be held so that he . . . should cry out, for this will make the rectum project out more." Thankfully, we have no illustration for this example. You're welcome. Afterward, he recommended a poultice of lentils and vegetables applied to the anus. Oh well. Cross lentil soup off the list of things you'll be eating this week.

We can also thank Hippocrates for inspiring generations of medical practitioners to reach for sizzling hot pokers. One of his famous aphorisms in the Corpus praises cautery as a panacea that doctors should try when other options didn't work: "As many conditions as drugs do not cure, the knife

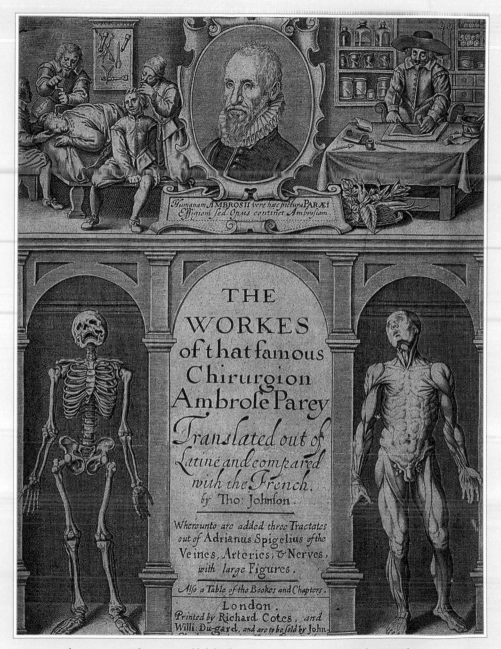

Ambroise Paré, French surgeon, tackled the "horride symptomes" of cautery in the sixteenth century.

cures; as many as a knife does not cure, fire cures; as many as fire does not cure, these have to be considered incurable."

In the first century, Celsus really took this "fire cures everything curable" theory and ran with it. He noted, "All afflictions . . . when inveterate, scarce admit a cure without cauterization." A cautery iron could be applied to the head for headaches until the skin ulcerated. Got a bad cough? Cautery should be used under the chin, on the neck, on the breasts, and below the shoulder blades. Epilepsy? Apoplexy? Cauterize the crap out of that poor patient.

With the invention of the gun, doctors were faced with a new and deadly problem that Hippocrates knew nothing about: bullet wounds. The ancient founding fathers of medicine didn't have to deal with guns, so practitioners in the fifteenth and sixteenth centuries had to wing it. Indeed, desperate times called for guesswork and boiling oil—until Ambroise Paré came on the scene.

At the tender age of twenty-seven and not yet sworn in as a surgeon, Paré was deployed during the third war between France and the Holy Roman Emperor, Charles V, in 1537. He dealt with gunshot wounds according to

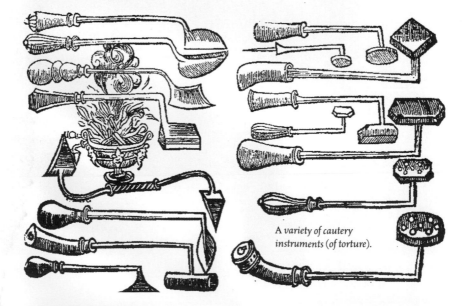

A variety of cautery instruments (of torture).

ST. HUBERT'S KEY

Let's say you get mauled by a rabid Chihuahua. We get it, you're having a bad day. Rabies is practically incurable, after all. But before you start glamorously foaming at the mouth, and because you have nothing to lose, how about you shove a burning hot nail into your wound?

The idea harkens back to the first century CE, when Celsus prescribed actual cautery for curing mad dog bites. And if you were *really* serious about burning the rabies out, you'd reach for a replica of St. Hubert's key.

The tool looked like a nail on steroids and was named after a first-century Belgian who was the patron saint of hunters, mathematicians, opticians, and metalworkers. (Random, but then again, David Lee Roth ended up as a paramedic, so . . .) Apparently, after St. Peter gave him the key, St. Hubert used it to cure a case of rabies, making him famous. For centuries afterward, people fashioned replicas of the tool, claiming that a burning hot St. Hubert's key could prevent rabies if it cauterized the wound of a dog bite. A good thought, except the rabies treatment also included cutting the bitten person's perfectly unbitten forehead, putting in a thread from St. Hubert's clothes, and covering the wound with a black cloth. The keys were even hung in houses for protection. Unfortunately, the superstition extended to the point where dogs and people were branded as a preventative measure, to stave off rabies.

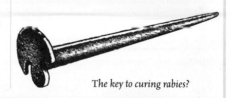

The key to curing rabies?

the writings of famous surgeons Hieronymus Brunschwig and Giovanni da Vigo—by cauterizing the wounds because the gunpowder was believed to be poisonous.

But Paré had a little problem. He ran out of elderberry oil for cauterization. Instead, he used the post-cauterization recipe of egg yolk, rose oil, and turpentine on the wounds and went to bed, terrified that the wounded soldiers would all be dead in the morning. He awoke to a surprise—the cauterized patients had horrible, oozy, excruciating wounds, but the ones that weren't cauterized were recovering painlessly. So much for the "poisoned gunshot wound" theory. Paré started to doubt the long-standing practice, noting cautery caused "horride symptoms . . . and oft times death it selfe."

Paré's discovery was a landmark, but practitioners weren't throwing out their oil and irons just yet. Cautery was still used for gunshot wounds and amputations more than two hundred years later during the American Civil War. Despite the fact that Paré showed that ligating vessels (tying them closed) worked better in amputations, wartime dictated cheap, fast, and easy methods. Sadly, that list didn't include painless ones.

Counterintuitively, it was the pain of cautery that made it so popular for some. Let us introduce you to the baffling concept of counterirritation.

BURN THIS, NOT THAT: COUNTERIRRITATION

In 1882, a troubled patient consulted Dr. A. R. Carman of New York. The young woman had been bedridden for weeks. She couldn't gainfully work in her position as a teacher and was rendered useless by violent headaches, crippling insomnia, and that useful catchall term for when everything simply feels awful—*malaise*. Sure, pharmacies were full of treatments that might have helped—tonics to pep up the spirit and liven up the liver, sedative draughts to ease the sufferer into a nice drugged sleep or an afternoon stupor—but Dr. Carman had a better idea. Similar patients had a miraculous recovery after receiving a series of burns up and down the spine.

So how did she do? Well, she also experienced an astounding recovery after her cautery treatments and went right back to work. In hindsight, it's clear that there may have been other factors at play. (If someone threatened to sear you with hot irons again if you stayed in bed for another day, wouldn't you jump up and run back to work instead?) To doctors at the time, though, it was a classic case study in the wonder of counterirritation via cautery.

Counterirritation, sometimes called counterstimulation, is not when you slap someone for saying something rude and receive a nice smack right back (actually, that would be double counterirritation and an invitation for a lawsuit). The theory went that if you provide a source of irritation or stimulation apart from where the actual problem is, it draws the offending sickness elsewhere so the original area can heal. Books are full of anecdotes, like the fellow with the "frenzies" (thought to be brain irritation) cured "by casual application of fire to the lower parts." Casual? How is that casual?

But sometimes, the theory seemed a little too soft in the face of the obvious. In 1875, Dr. Charles-Édouard Brown-Séquard used cautery to "wake people up" from deep comas (which technically wouldn't work—he probably just woke sleeping patients). Counterirritation via cautery was also used to treat melancholy and suspected werewolfism "when all other remedies fail." Practitioners claimed it even cured headaches, sunstroke, and paralysis.

Surely, though, cautery imparted a hefty placebo effect, or at least distraction from the actual problem. In 1610, Jacques Ferrand recommended cauterizing the forehead with a searing-hot iron for lovesickness. For swelling, a twelfth-century physician recommended no less than twenty burns all over the body, including the temples, chest, ankles, under the lip, collarbones, hips. . . . You get the idea.

It shouldn't be surprising that counterirritation wasn't exactly a hit with patients. Dr. Carman had one final note about cautery that pretty much says it all: "It is sometimes difficult to convince a timid person that it is not a terrible procedure."

Agreed. But fire wasn't even the worst of it. Some antiquated methods of counterirritation and counterstimulation were blisteringly awful. And we mean *blistering*.

BLISTERING: A BEETLE TALE

Now let's say you chose option 3 from those headache cure options. Perhaps you found putting a red-hot iron on someone's back to get her out of bed a little tame? Then you'll be pleased to meet *Lytta vesicatoria*, a type of blister beetle, also known as Spanish fly.

PEAS, ANYONE?

Sometimes, blistering or cautery wasn't enough to draw out the problem. The more bad humors that could pour out of a wound, the better, right? So on occasion, the blister was unroofed or a cautery iron was used to create a small divot in the skin. A dried pea was then shoved inside. The pea would cause more irritation, hopefully producing copious pus. (The authors would now like to apologize for your inability to eat peas in the forthcoming weeks.)

Occasionally, the pea was replaced or supplemented by a *seton*, a thread that was needled through the skin, preferably in the back of the neck. The thread—made more irritating with a coating of resin-based salve—would then be "flossed" daily through the new wound. Basically, it was like putting rosin on a violin bow and playing a wound. The accompanying sound must have been pretty awful. Just think of all that squishy pus, not to mention the human wailing.

Spanish fly's reputation as an aphrodisiac is well known, but its usage as a blistering agent goes back centuries. The beetle is quite a pretty thing—half an inch in length, with an iridescent green back. Better to look and not touch, though: Its body contains a compound called cantharidin, which causes blistering when applied to the skin. The males of the species have more cantharidin than the females. They usually offer a romantic package of cantharidin-laced secretions to wrap around the female's eggs to keep them safe from predators.

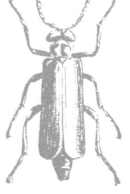

Spanish fly, at your service.

A London dispensary from the early 1800s offered a recipe containing a pound of beetle powder, a pound of wax, and a pound of lard. Toothsome. This paste was applied to the skin for as long as it took to form a blister. Where? It depended. Generally, the aim was to blister near the problem in order to draw it to the surface. So the abdomen was blistered for stomach ailments, or the lower legs for gout. If the patient became delirious, he would be blistered on the head instead. Unfortunately for some, the blisters caused gangrene, where the underlying flesh simply died and blackened.

Why blister? An 1845 medical textbook describes a leading theory from a Dr. Charles Williams: Many illnesses, like the measles, didn't improve until after the skin erupted. Instead of a symptom, the rash was thought to be the actual pathway to healing. Hence, countless healers thought that irritating the skin could cure, and these theories went back as far as ancient Greek physicians.

And the bigger the blister, the better. Blistering agents—known as vesicants—were as plentiful as Jelly Belly flavors. Tartar emetic, an antimony compound typically used to cause vomiting (see Antimony, page 15), was also applied as an ointment to produce pus-filled blisters that resembled smallpox. Strong acids were effective but messy and hard to control. Same with jets of boiling water; boiling oil worked, too. Both made nice, painful blisters via partial-thickness burns.

Like most quack cures, blistering was used as a last-resort treatment for just about everything: hysteria, laryngitis, hypochondria, inflammation, fevers, diphtheria, encephalitis, even opiate addiction as late as 1929. Then what? Well, sometimes the blisters were sliced open to allow continuous draining of fluids, or blistering ointments were used to create a crop of blisters to maintain a "constant drain of . . . humours," according to an eighteenth-century English materia medica. Sometimes, the fluids were collected, and in a rarely used process called phlyctenotherapy, the blister liquid was bizarrely injected back into the patient.

Blisters not your thing? Smart choice. I guess you finally decided option 4 was really the way to go. World peace, FTW.

Blistering and Cautery Today

Cautery continues today, though it is decidedly less awful a procedure. Partly because we've got anesthesia to thank, and partly because we've abandoned humoral theory and no longer panic in our helplessness when faced with disease. Surgeons wield modern electrocautery instruments with precision. Ye olde hot irons have long since been left to cool in museums around the world.

People still employ a type of distraction and counterirritation by rubbing on salves with menthol, capsaicin, camphor, or methyl salicylate (with the telltale wintergreen scent) for body pain or congestion. These salves tend to cause slight tingling and burning sensations of varying degrees, but do not get absorbed in sufficient amounts to precisely target that phlegmy airway or aching shoulder.

As for blistering, there is a good reason why it has no place in modern toolboxes. Blistering cannot truly "draw out" a disease from the body. And it's obvious why the gentler distractions of medicated muscle salves are on the shelves, instead of Spanish fly ointments. Modern patches and rubs actually do feel nice, so long as you're not covering ginormous patches of skin with the medicines (yes, you can actually be poisoned to death by those minty-smelling rubs). They are relatively safe, and happily there won't be a bubbling, drippy, oozy blister in sight.

15

Enemas & Clysters

Of Autointoxication, Pfear of Ptomaine, Public Enemas, a Rectal Blasting Cushion, and Guardians of the Anus

On this earth, right now, there exists an eight-hundred-pound enema bulb. Yes. It's a brass statue situated in the spa town of Zheleznovodsk in Russia, famous for its colonics. The enema bulb is about four feet in length and held aloft by three cherubic angels, who aim it lovingly toward the sky. It's as if they're temptingly inviting some celestial buttocks down to earth for a nice anal washout. What a gilded tribute and testament to our obsession with the enema!

Since the beginning of recorded time, humans have been fixated on their bowels. Medical practitioners have always battled the beast called constipation, and their sword in this fight has often been the enema. Sure, constipation is a nagging problem that no one wants, but enemas were thought to cure all sorts of problems besides sluggish stools.

The word *enema* originates from a Greek word meaning "to throw" or "send in." Later, the Latin meaning became synonymous with enemas: inject. The seventeenth-century term for enema was *clyster*, perhaps a somewhat prettier word, which sprouted from the Greek word for "wash."

Throughout history, enemas have contained a range of agents, including water, herbal concoctions, milk, molasses, turpentine, honey, beer, soaps, wine, and oils. What did they treat? Just as colorful a range of ailments—tuberculosis, dropsy, hernias, appendicitis, depression, poor nutrition, headaches (Mozart's father once famously said—"the arse cures the head"), obesity, sluggishness, breathing problems, fever-borne illnesses, sexual dysfunction, drowning, and coughing up blood. Somewhere in that rear cave of the ailment-addled human was a dark place that promised health, if it was simply power-washed with a deft hand.

The delivery system started out as more rudimentary, with hollowed gourds, tube-shaped bones, or animal bladders. Thoughtfully, some people were employed as "blowers" to give the medicated liquids a little oral push to their dark destinations. In more recent centuries, there were beautifully constructed clyster syringes of metal and

Spanish vase, c. 1600s. The inscription states, "I am Don Joaquin Hernandez's jar. Through intense devotion to my constitution I find myself on this occasion shamefully syringed at the hands of a serf."

ivory up to a foot long, or tubes with decorated pumping chambers, or chairs you sat on that shot the liquid . . . upstream. Most people might recognize the designs of rubber sacks with flexible tubing and rubberized enema bulbs that still exist today.

The range of products and medicated liquids was vast. The most famous and infamous have used them (Hitler used chamomile tea, not to drink, but as enemas for "cleansing" and possibly weight loss). So why the obsession with enemas?

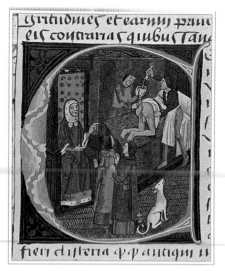

Galen administers a clyster. The dog seems rather entertained!

AUTOINTOXICATION: No, It's Not Drinking a Gallon of Beer

Much of the lure of enemas was due to the concept of autointoxication, the theory that feces are full of toxins and noxious agents. We now know that our own bowels don't naturally intoxicate us, but it took a few millennia to figure that out.

The ancient Egyptians had called it *wḥdw*, a putrefactive element found in feces that caused disease, and therefore purged the body via emetics and enemas for three days a month, according to Herodotus's writings in the fifth century BCE. Hippocrates, around the same time, was reported to have said that disease arose from the vapors produced by undigested food in the colon.

In the second century, Galen thought that the body's humors would putrefy given the right conditions, and expelling them in the feces helped. Then there was the theory that these putrefaction particles might be in the air, ready to cause disease. In addition to originating inside the bowels, these "miasmas" were thought to be disease-carrying airs that came from fetid swamps or rotting vegetation. Also simply called bad air or night air, miasmas were blamed as a cause of many epidemics, including cholera and the Black Death. This concept was widely accepted for centuries. In *Jane Eyre*, the typhus that killed half of the orphans grew from "fog and fog-bred pestilence." Ma Ingalls in *Little House on the Prairie* cautioned Pa against eating watermelon because "it grew in the night air" and might give him the "fever 'n' ague" (ague being malaria, itself from the Italian for "bad air") that was striking down settlers. Pa ate the watermelon anyway and survived.

It's easy to understand why constipation was a theoretical source of putrefaction—human waste, to most people, is utterly revolting, and knowing that disgusting pile of crap came from inside you, well, it must mean that excrement itself is a perilous thing. Perhaps if feces spent longer amounts of time in the colon and bowel movements happened infrequently, then these dirty toxins would escape into the body. The putrefactive elements would then be absorbed into the circulation, causing fever and pus, insanity, and hemorrhage, then world wars, then alien invasions. . . . You get the idea.

In the 1700s, Johann Kämpf loudly proclaimed that all illness came from impacted feces (dry, hard stool that is "stuck" in the colon). Hence, if you expelled them faster with enemas, you were less likely to get sick.

Or so the theory goes.

In the 1800s, the feverish fear regarding "ptomaines" worsened these beliefs about the evil lurking within our bowels. Ptomaines are the chemicals—putrescine and cadaverine (tasty names!)— that make rotting things smell bad and were thought to be the particles that caused severe sickness. Basically, the assumption was that germs consumed organic matter in your intestine, and ptomaines were the by-product. From the Greek word *ptōma* for "fallen body" or "corpse," ptomaines were blamed for any and every food-borne illness. Not only were they inaccurately considered to cause food poisoning, ptomaines were also thought to arise in a constipated feces. (Autointoxication strikes again!) This added to the fear that inner feces alone made people sick, instead of being the end product of a healthy physiologic process. Rectal cleanliness could fix it all, for if filth was the root cause of disease (true, in many cases), then internal colonic cleanliness could prevent it. One little problem, though—the ptomaine theory was wrong. Bacteria and their toxins, not ptomaines, actually cause food poisoning, so the theory fell out of use. Washing hands? A great way to prevent infections. Washing colons? Not so much.

In addition to autointoxication was the pervasive humoral theory. For multiple centuries, "clyster, bleed, purge" was the treatment for everything, particularly if the black bile/melancholic humor was out of sorts. Methods of cure that made bile flow out the anus ruled. The clyster was looked upon as a rectal savior for all things awry in the human body. The love of enemas became so extreme that Molière's *The Imaginary Invalid* poked fun at it in 1673. When the doctor is asked repeatedly how to cure dropsy, then diseased lungs, then chronic illnesses, his response is always "Give a clyster, then bleed the patient, afterward purge him. Rebleed him, repurge him, and reclyster him."

The scene is a funny and sharp-tongued editorial on current medicine and its one-size-fits-all cures that lasted for far too long.

CHAMPIONS OF THE RECTAL DOOR

In ancient Egypt, concern about health and digestion was so paramount that the enema was an indispensable part of life. Documents from 1600 to 1550 BCE described enemas and how the pharaohs had their own specialized health-care servant—the honorably named "Guardian of the Anus." We might laugh at this idea, but unlike today, the health of the lower digestive tract in ancient Egypt was appreciated with far less comedic flair.

Hippocrates also touted the benefits of the beloved enema, for "ardent fevers" or intermittent fevers often seen with malaria. If that didn't work, "then purge with the boiled milk of asses." Galen, in the second century CE, described his ministrations to a sick lady coughing up blood. Aside from rubbing her body and giving her opium, "I ordered a sharp clyster." Ouch.

In the Middle Ages, we first begin seeing artistic renderings of clyster and enema use. There's a fifteenth-century illustration of Galen pouring fluids down a funnel into someone's rectum while others mill about in the room. Nearby, a dog is howling, or laughing; it's rather unclear.

Clysters had become de rigueur and à la mode in fifteenth- and sixteenth-century France—perhaps because royalty loved them so. King Louis XIV was rumored to have enjoyed two thousand treatments in his lifetime. *Two thousand.* At the height of the craze in France, many used clysters as often as three

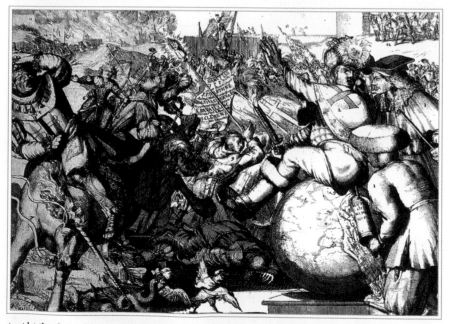

Amidst the chaos of the seventeenth-century Protestant rebellions, Louis XIV receives a clyster while sitting on the world.

times per day to "maintain health." The ordinariness of the procedure was illustrated famously by the Duchess of Burgundy. She had her servant duck beneath her skirts to administer a clyster. *In front of the king.* Naturally, she was modestly covered while the clyster was given. But it makes you rather glad you weren't part of the royal court of Louis XIV or one of the servants in charge of clysters—no matter how blinged-out those syringes were.

DIY ENEMAS

In the late 1800s, shysters started to exploit our fears of autointoxication with an array of products. Alcinous Burton Jamison sold his "eager colon cleanser" as well as his horseshoe-shaped "internal fountain bath," all while trying to scare his customers about the "pest-house of absorbed poison" within the intestines. Eager patients were strapped down onto tilting tables like the "West Gravitiser," in an effort to keep things moving in the right direction— down and out. Or consider "Dr. Young," whose treatments went, well, the other direction. His "self-retaining rectal dilators" (see Sex, page 244) were short, phallus-shaped rods of increasing size, touted to cure constipation and hemorrhoids. Because nothing soothes hemorrhoid pains like sticking a thick rubber rod up your behind.

We'll now take a brief interlude to meet Dr. Charles A. Tyrrell (1843– 1918), who perhaps wears the crown of quackery for his constipation wares. The story begins with him telling his own story, of course. He claimed that before his medical career, he'd traveled to exotic locales including New Zealand, South Africa, and the Far East; he'd dined with indigenous peoples and experienced diseases like "jungle fever" (malaria), typhoid fever, and dys- entery. He was also paralyzed by a gunshot wound in India. But it wasn't until 1880 when a second bout of paralysis struck, for unknown reasons, that ene- mas came to the rescue. He read a treatise by a physician extolling the cure- all nature of the enema. After years of self-treatment and a recovery from the paralysis, he had a proctological epiphany. Tyrrell opened the Hygienic Institute in New York City and announced, "There is only one cause for disease," and it was constipation.

Enemas to the rescue! (Cue the trumpets!)

Continuing with the autointoxication theories of yore, Tyrrell believed that illnesses such as seizures, achy joints, cholera, and dysentery were due to the rotting miasmas arising from the gut, so extreme measures were necessary to flush them out. Most enema bags at the time consisted of a rubber bag filled with liquid that used gravity to insert its contents into a reclined patient, via a tube and nozzle. But Tyrrell's "J. B. L. Cascade" was different. J. B. L. stood for "joy, beauty, life" and promised to provide an "internal bath," via a large rubber bottle that held five quarts of liquid. A nozzle protruded out of the center, so a health-seeker could impale his- or herself on it while in a seated position. The person's weight would compress the reservoir and blast their innards, as often as they pleased. He recommended the Cascade up to four times a week and was happy to promote his wares using quotes from satisfied customers. One man's wife saved the Cascade—and only the Cascade—from a house fire. Hopefully, they had no children. Another gentleman gifted his daughter a Cascade for her wedding. How loving and utterly gross. Sadly for us, it's not available on the wedding registries at Bed Bath & Beyond.

Later in the twentieth century, German-born physician Max Gerson continued the crusade of detoxification and made a tidy profit. Early in his career, a plant-based diet had ended his migraines, and he claimed it cured a pesky bout of skin tuberculosis. He blamed environmental pollutants in the body. In the 1920s, he proposed that cancer, too,

A cure for hemorrhoids? Nope.

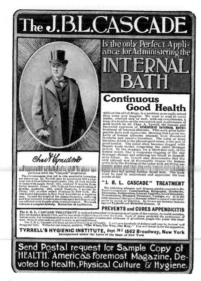

"Joy, Beauty, Life," via an enema blast.

could be cured, and recommended vegetable juices, vitamins, pancreatic enzymes, coffee and castor-oil enemas, plus rectal ozone gas treatments. Why use a coffee enema? Apparently, it helped detoxify the liver (which it doesn't, really).

Gerson ended up dying under mysterious circumstances his daughter claims that he was poisoned by arsenic. Nevertheless, the Gerson Institute still touts its claims and plenty of people are willing to believe in coffee enemas' effectiveness. Fill it to the rim with a nice cuppa joe? If only Starbucks had it on their drive-through menu.

ENEMAS TODAY: THE REAR ENDING

The idea of autointoxication is hard to kill. Today, people continue to receive high colonics in the name of "detoxing" despite the facts. Since constipation can actually be helped (though not necessarily cured) with enemas, they are a mainstay in the medical world and are available everywhere. The rectum and lower colon have the ability to absorb fluids and medications, hence the existence of suppository medicine. What has changed, however, is *why* we legitimately give enemas.

Humoral medicine and "bleed, purge, and clyster" are no longer considered scientifically accurate ways to treat diseases now that we have a firmer understanding of their causes. The idea of ptomaines fell from public consciousness because most people accept that food poisoning occurs from pathogens such as *Salmonella* and *E. coli*.

In 1912, Dr. Arthur J. Cramp wrote a piece in *JAMA* that skewered Tyrrell and his Cascade. Tyrrell's professional testimonials were barely legitimate, written by nonphysician patent medicine makers or those who were conveniently dead at the time. Tyrrell called himself a physician when he started the Hygienic Institute, though it was years later, in his late fifties, when he received a medical degree from the dubious Eclectic Institute. It wasn't exactly Harvard.

And in 1919, a *JAMA* article by Dr. Walter C. Alvarez debunked autointoxication once and for all. He railed at physicians who ignored high blood pressure, uterine tumors, and kidney disease and focused solely on constipation as the cause of everything. Alvarez noted that the intestinal wall wasn't some porous open door to toxins and that the flora of the colon were beneficial, not harmful. A physician needed to listen to reason before "inoculating his patients with fear" and to disregard the "ready surgeons who have short-circuited a few colons."

Even so, the concept of removing toxins and "cleansing" via the bowels remains a billion-dollar industry, thanks to word-of-mouth, testimonials, and excellent marketing. One could say that the colon remains as much in the consciousness of the human race as it ever has.

Gerson's idea of using coffee enemas for cancer is also still an actively practiced treatment regimen by alternative therapists, despite a National Institutes of Health study showing that patients with pancreatic cancer lived longer with conventional chemotherapy. There will always be supporters of the coffee enema.

But please, for the love of Hippocrates, don't use boiling-hot coffee.

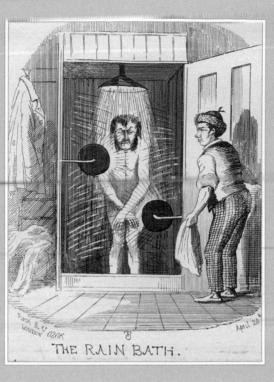

16

THE RAIN BATH.

Hydropathy & the Cold Water Cure

Of Austrian Badasses, Water Cure Establishments, and a Surprising Number of Ways to Get Drenched in Cold Water

Vincenz Priessnitz was only eight years old when his father went blind in 1807. When that tragedy was followed four years later by the death of his older brother, it left Vincenz the primary caregiver for the family and their farm in the Austrian alps.

One day, when Priessnitz was eighteen years old, he was driving a cart loaded down with oats to a neighboring farm when his horse startled. He jumped down to calm the horse, but the animal kicked out its hind legs, knocking out his front teeth and throwing him directly in front of the cart, which promptly rolled over him. The boy passed out from the pain of multiple broken ribs and significant internal damage.

When he awoke, under the care of a visiting surgeon, Priessnitz was declared a likely goner. With luck, the attending surgeon thought he might live but would certainly be an invalid for the rest of his life.

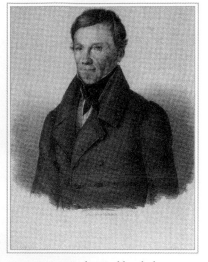

Vincenz Priessnitz, dressing like a badass.

Vincenz Priessnitz, however, was a dyed-in-the-wool Austrian badass. He wasn't going to give up so easily. After tossing aside the surgeon's hot compresses around his broken ribs, which were just increasing his pain, Priessnitz got up from bed, set a wooden chair against his abdomen, took a deep breath, and . . . pushed (pausing here for a collective gasp).

And it worked. The teenager literally set his own ribs back into place, freeing up the terrible pressure on his internal organs.

While lying in bed recovering from being a badass, Priessnitz recalled a scene in the woods one afternoon where he observed a deer return several times to a cold spring to bathe a wound. Applying the same logic to his current situation, he began treating his injuries with a series of compresses made of linen towels soaked in cold water, a sharp contrast with the hot water compresses advocated by his physician. He also began drinking large amounts of cold water and regularly changing his bandages.

As a result, perhaps predictably to modern-day audiences, Priessnitz staved off infection, prevented fever from taking root, and had himself sufficiently cured of his injuries to be up and about supervising farm work just a few days after the accident.

Although he didn't yet realize it, Priessnitz had also just discovered the "cold water cure," a phenomenon that would soon sweep the medical community of the early nineteenth century and make him a wealthy and famous man.

MAKE YOURSELF UNCOMFORTABLE

Today, we would largely regard Priessnitz's medical conclusions as common sense. Drink lots of water? Check. Regularly change your bandages? Check. Clean your wounds? Check. But in the world of his youth, none of these practices were yet accepted as commonplace.

Priessnitz rebuilt his house into a sanitarium, dubbed the Gräfenburg Water Cure, in 1826. News spread fast through the Austrian Alps of a boy who had brought himself back from the brink of death, a healer who could cure illness and injury with cold water.

Priessnitz's popularity and success rate were phenomenal, which more than anything gives us insight into the appalling sanitary conditions of early nineteenth-century Europe. Imagine the days when you could make a successful career as a physician by simply advising people to take a few more baths. Soon Priessnitz even had European royalty lining up to take a turn at the Gräfenburg Water Cure.

Imitators sprang up all over Europe. In England, numerous water cures—there dubbed "hydropathic institutes"—opened for business, attracting attention and glowing reviews from a variety of Victorian luminaries such as Thomas Carlyle, Charles Dickens, and Alfred Lord Tennyson.

Each hydropathic institute was basically a slight variation on a common theme: Bathe more often and drink more water. Specific techniques varied,

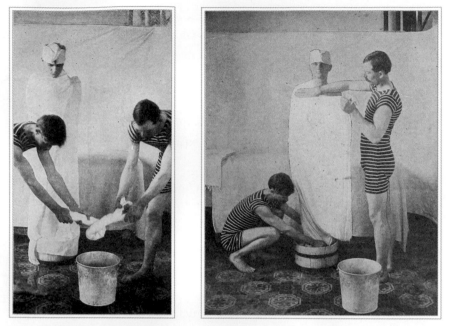

Rub-a-dub-dub...

however, from place to place. Although the concepts of bathing and hydrating are sound, like so many quack treatments, the water cure often took its good ideas to uncomfortable and dangerous proportions. Here are some of the water cure methods you would find at hydropathic institutes in the nineteenth century:

Wet sheet In a treatment seemingly inspired by the symptoms that fever victims endure, a patient was wrapped tightly in a sheet soaked with cold water, then instructed to lie down. After the sheet dried, the patient would begin to sweat profusely from the constricting body wrap. Eventually, the sheet was removed and the patient was dumped into a pool of cold

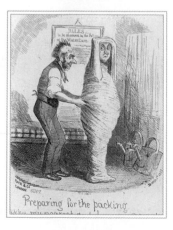

Preparing for the packing

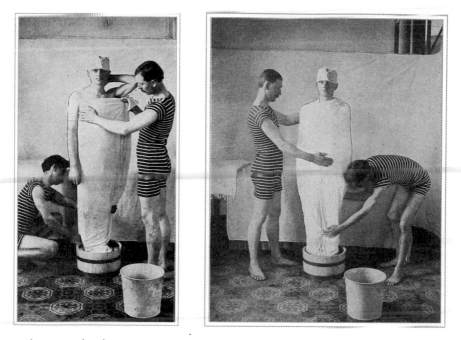

. . . three men and a tub.

water, followed by a rigorous drying. This cold-hot-cold treatment was a good way to stay awake, but probably not the best idea if you were sick with a cold, or a fever, or really pretty much anything at all.

Wet dress A loose-fitting nightgown, soaked in cold water, was worn by the patient as he or she walked about the institute, thus first introducing to fashion the perennially popular "wet T-shirt look." (Happily, to conform to Victorian standards of propriety, there were separate wings for men and women.) Sometimes patients even slept in a wet dress. This billowing dress became so popular in the confining age of corsets and petticoats that it led to an entirely new women's fashion statement: bloomers (so named for journalist Amelia Bloomer, who wrote passionately and frequently about the streetwear version of the wet dress introduced by Elizabeth Smith and Elizabeth Cady Stanton). The only real benefit to wearing a wet dress was the

CHARLES DARWIN

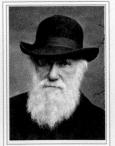

Charles Darwin was an enthusiastic adopter of the water cure. The scientist suffered all his life from a mysterious, undiagnosed ailment with a bizarre array of symptoms. As a result, Darwin spent much of his time trying new medical developments, including hydrotherapy. (Note: After the topic baffled medical historians for many years, many experts now conclude that Darwin suffered from Crohn's disease.)

Darwin wrote of his treatment at a hydropathic institute: "I cannot in the least understand how hydropathy can act as it certainly does on me. It dulls one's brain splendidly, I have not thought about a single species of any kind since leaving home."

High praise indeed from someone obsessed with the evolution of species.

refreshing break for your body from the crushing confines of a corset. As for being cold and wet? That was just an obstacle for your body to overcome so you could enjoy that free-flowing dress.

Cold shower This practice, familiar to today's reader, was quite a shock to the nineteenth-century water cure patient. Remember this was the era of "I think I bathed sometime last January, so I'm still good for a while." Not exactly a showering culture. Some hydropathic institutes plumbed in cold river water to plunge down onto patients from a height of at least ten feet above their heads, a practice that literally flattened some poor bathers onto the ground. In winter (and water cure establishments didn't break for the winter, by the way), patients also had to dodge falling icicles. Surviving the cold shower treatment at a hydropathic institute was really its own accomplishment.

Cold water enema Self-explanatory.

The Power of Shock

While the treatments patients encountered at hydropathic institutes were often uncomfortable, they were at the very least voluntary. You could come and go as you wished. Those simple freedoms of choice and movement, however, were not luxuries enjoyed by the patients at insane asylums in the eighteenth and early nineteenth centuries, where they were repeatedly doused with cold water or nearly drowned in baths in attempts to generate fear or "correct" behavior.

As the nineteenth century progressed, a comparatively enlightened viewpoint descended upon the asylum physicians, who began to use hydrotherapy in a non-punitive manner. Or at least that's how they felt about it. Asylum physicians started employing a variety of hydropathic techniques to calm patients, "shock" the madness out of their brains, or relieve the seemingly feverish heat of insanity. The patients, however, probably felt like the following hydropathic techniques were pretty damn punitive:

Cold water pour Recommended by Dr. Benjamin Rush, the "Father of American Psychiatry," the cold water pour attempted to "establish governance over the deranged patients" by dumping streams of cold water down their coat sleeves.

Continuous hot bath Imagine being trapped in a hot tub you can't escape. The patient was lowered into a tub with a continuous flow of water kept between 95 and 110 degrees. The tub was then covered with a sheet that had a hole in it for the patient to stick his head through. The patient was kept in the tub for anywhere from a few hours to a few weeks. A Swedish nurse recollected the treatment: "Patients could live in there for three weeks at a time in the bath. They slept in the bathtubs too. We fed them in the bath and held the drinking glass up to their mouths. . . . They peed and defecated in the water, of course. . . . Some patients became calmer from it, they really did! It exhausted them."

Douche A different type of douche than what just popped into your mind. This douche was a stream of cold water falling continuously on the head of a restrained patient. It was greatly feared, often producing faintness, vomiting, physical exhaustion, and shock.

Pelvic douche A high-pressure water jet aimed at the genitals, and a much more pleasant alternative to the "douche" technique listed above. The "pelvic douche" was employed to cure all manner of "women's disorders" such as the pervasive hysteria diagnosis that ran rampant in the nineteenth century. The goal, of course, was to obtain the euphoric benefits of an orgasm, although no one involved in pelvic douches would have called it that at the time. Writing in 1843, a French physician described the popularity of the pelvic douche among his female patients: "The reaction of the organism

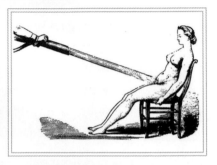

to the cold, which causes the skin to flush, and the reestablishment of equilibrium [author's note: best orgasm euphemism ever] all create for many persons so agreeable a sensation that it is necessary to take precautions that they do not go beyond the prescribed time, which is usually four or five minutes."

Drenching Remember taking part in the ice bucket challenge in 2014 that raised a lot of money for ALS? Drenching was basically an involuntary ice bucket challenge, not for a good cause, and repeated ad nauseam. (Literally.)

Dripping machine A bucket positioned above a patient's head would drip slowly and steadily onto a specific spot on the patient's forehead. And yep, this is the exact same technique more commonly labeled "Chinese water torture" (although, to be fair, that was supposedly invented by an Italian sometime in the fifteenth or sixteenth century).

EIGHT GLASSES? TRY THIRTY.

Vigorously ingesting cold water was one of the signature treatments at a water cure institute. Our modern medical advice to drink "eight glasses of water a day" originates from hydropathy treatments, although it's a bit more moderate in its amount. At one water institute, a patient reported drinking thirty glasses of water—before breakfast!

Of course, it was inevitable that some quacks would take a good idea, like drinking water, and push it to excess. Enter Dr. Fereydoon Batmanghelidj, whose popular book *Your Body's Many Cries for Water* came out in 1992. Batmanghelidj claimed that dehydration was the cause of "many painful degenerative diseases, asthma, allergies, hypertension, excess body weight, and some emotional problems, including depression." The cure? Drink water. A lot of water.

Batmanghelidj claimed for himself a compelling origin story: While the physician was a political prisoner in Iran, he was often instructed by the guards to treat his fellow inmates. Lacking proper medical tools, the doctor turned to the only thing available to him: water. He concluded that pain is really the body's way of calling out for more water. So water became Batmanghelidj's cure for, well, basically everything.

The physician's science, however, was a bit off. He claimed in his book that water was a main source of energy for the brain and the body by producing "hydro-electric" energy, which is totally baseless. He also claimed an extensive background in medical research, a background that was mysteriously elusive when other physicians attempted to check his credentials. And the connection between drinking water and curing the pantheon of diseases claimed in his book has no scientific basis at all.

Nevertheless, Batmanghelidj's book was a bestseller in the 1990s and remains in print, and popular, today.

MINERAL WATER

The twenty-first-century bottled water trend, a $15 billion industry in 2015, also has its origins in nineteenth-century medicine. In the later part of the 1800s, Americans drank gallons of mineral water from more than 500 springs around the country. Their goal was to be cured of all manner of diseases, but most particularly that general catch-all *nervous exhaustion*, a term better understood now as *stress*.

Mineral water grew in popularity as a general belief spread that minerals naturally occurring in spring water were curative and a much better choice for drinking than gross city water. (Considering the general state of city cleanliness in the late nineteenth century, they probably had a good point.) Doctors recommended that patients drink mineral water during the "inactive phase" of the disease, at the rate of about two to four glasses per day.

The medical claims about mineral water, however, were not actually based on scientific evidence, and mineral water manufacturers drew the ire of the American Medical Association, which issued a damning report in 1918: "No mineral water will be accepted by the medical profession for alleged medicinal properties supported only by testimonials from bucolic statesmen and romantic old ladies." Ouch. Bottled mineral water fell out of fashion as a result, but resurfaced again in the 1980s when Americans were suffering a collective hangover after the decade-long binge of alcohol drinking between 1970 and 1980. Bottled mineral water became a popular alternative to a stiff drink at the end of the night. And the practice has stuck with us ever since.

In the wake of Batmanghelidj came the Millennium Oxygen Cooler, which debuted in the early 2000s with effusive claims to oxygenate your water. The cooler boasted a 600 percent higher concentration of oxygen than your average, run-of-the-mill tap water. The proclaimed benefits of these elevated levels included providing more oxygen to the blood cells "to enhance the body's ability to fight infectious bacteria, microbes, and viruses." The oxygenated water would even clean out "excreta and those toxins left in the body." The manufacturer even included the bizarre claim that the oxygen level in the air today is "far less than in ancient times (oxygen content was at 38 percent ten thousand years ago compared with the 21 percent it is now)."

In a panic yet? Don't be. The oxygen content of the earth's atmosphere is about the same as it was ten thousand years ago. And your body can't extract oxygen from water, even if it were beneficial to do so. Humans aren't fish. If you want to take in more oxygen, try this simple suggestion instead: Take a deep breath.

THE WATER CURE TODAY

Many of the tenets of the water cure are still with us today. Regular bathing practices were first introduced by hydropathy, and few Americans in the twenty-first century would consider going a single day without taking a bath or shower. (To see how far we've come, here is an excerpt from a letter to the *Boston Moral Reformer* in 1835: "I have been in the habit during this past winter of taking a warm bath every three weeks. Is this too often to follow the year round?") Non-restrictive clothing has been adopted en masse. Modern spas—and the hydropathic therapies available at most gyms and athletic clubs—are direct descendants of the nineteenth-century hydropathic institutes. Drinking enough water every day is another universal given in modern medicinal practice, although the exact amount of water you should drink still attracts vigorous debate.

Despite the arrival of quacks on the water cure scene, the original hydropaths were on to something. They came along at just the right time in the progression of history to bring about much needed changes in personal hygiene. By drinking water, getting a lot of exercise, and taking regular baths, people could indeed prevent some diseases and lead healthier lives.

Next time you count out your water glasses for a given day, you're in effect participating in a nineteenth-century medical curiosity. Just don't dump buckets of cold water on your friend claiming that you're helping him cool the fire in his brain.

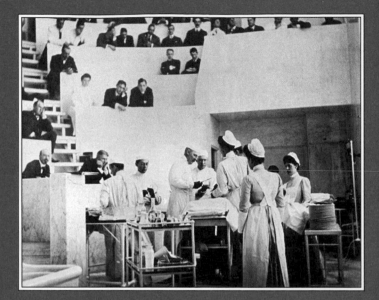

17

Surgery

Of Crossbow Scalpels, the Need for Speed,
300 Percent Mortality Rates, the Theater of Surgery,
and Pus-Covered Coats

Chances are you've had surgery. If not? Just wait. You probably will someday. What was once a limited discipline saved for the most extreme of medical ailments is now common. Elective, often. We assume all will be sterile and painless, that our surgeons will be skilled (and actually surgeons, duh). But once upon a pus-filled time, surgery was not so tidy and precise.

Surgery is breaking through the ultimate mortal barrier—the body itself. Slicing through skin, poking through eyeballs, sawing off bones, and ligating blood vessels means altering nature and the natural history of disease and trauma. Is it somewhat godlike? Eh, let's leave that answer to the psychoanalysts.

Since ancient times, doctors have turned to surgery for fixing broken bones, treating traumatic injuries, and cutting off diseased limbs. We've drilled holes in skulls for headaches and epilepsy, cauterized amputations with scalding irons, and even shot arrows back out of bodies. That's right. Arrow wounds were the chief problem from prehistoric times until the advent of

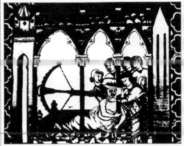

Shooting an arrow out of the patient's neck with a crossbow ... well, it seemed like a good idea at the time.

guns. Removing the arrow was a troublesome task, and on occasion, physicians thoughtfully decided that using a crossbow was the ideal method of removal. A medieval illustration shows a poor soul clinging to a pillar while the embedded arrow in his neck is attached to a crossbow to remove it. And you thought you were having a bad week.

Here, we'll be focusing on the dawn of modern surgery, beginning in the sixteenth century, when discovery, desperation, and ingenuity (and occasionally egos) all collided. In the grand, bloody, and smelly history of the operating room, there are several stopping points that leave us rather aghast. Through the lens of the present day, the annals of surgery are filled with scientifically unsound practices and charlatans. Let's scrub in and take a look.

Seventeenth-century German surgical instrument. Or evil scissors. You choose.

"Time Me, Gentlemen!"
The Costs of Speed and Showmanship

Amputation was perhaps the most common surgical procedure performed for thousands of years. In the face of leg wounds and deadly gangrene, it was often the best chance of survival, even if the mortality rate was as horrible as 60 percent or more (during the Franco-Prussian war in 1870, the mortality rate for amputations was a staggering 76 percent).

Until the nineteenth century, there was no reliable anesthesia, which meant that amputations had to be a quick affair to minimize the patient's waking nightmare. In the name of speed, often everything was cut at the same level, termed a *chop* or *guillotine* amputation. As if that term weren't

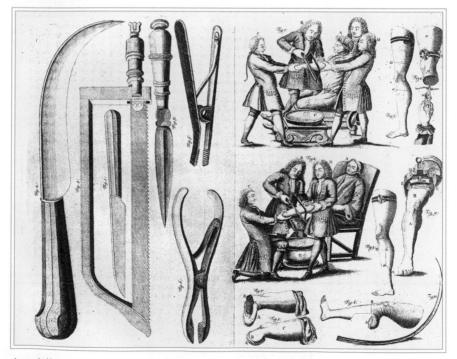

Amputation instruments and a helpful how-to.

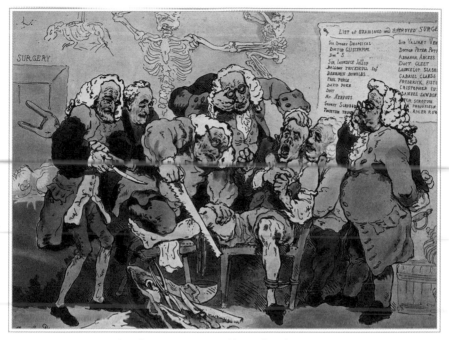

A *1793 amputation. Notice how the patient is restrained by people and ropes.*

horrible enough, in World War I, French surgeons called it amputation *en saucisson*, which likened the procedure to slicing a sausage in half. Tasty.

Although that might sound terrifying, if you were a badly wounded soldier, you would want a speedy sausage-chop, too. From the sixteenth to the nineteenth century, a typical leg amputation would go thusly: The patient was forcibly held down to prevent movement (and perhaps changing their mind and staggering away), while a tourniquet was applied to block off the main artery of the leg. Using a curved blade, the surgeon would cut skin and muscle around the bone, ideally in one single slice, and then saw the bone off. The open vessels would sometimes be cauterized (by hot irons, boiling oil, or chemically with vitriol), and the flesh was either left as is or sewn closed.

All this was done in less time than it takes to watch a YouTube music video. Eighteenth-century Scottish surgeon Benjamin Bell could amputate a thigh in six seconds. French surgeon Dominique Jean Larrey was comparatively slow. But in his defense, during the Napoleonic wars, he performed two hundred amputations in a twenty-four-hour period—one every seven minutes.

Sure, speed reduced the time the patient would spend in unendurable pain. But it also led to sloppy work. Often, bone was left protruding because the flesh withdrew from the cutting plane. Sliced flesh could be ragged, slowing the healing process. The speed of the procedure and awkward positioning to get around the limb meant accidental slices elsewhere. And no matter how fast the surgeon, operations were generally accompanied by the bloodcurdling screams of the patient.

Sometimes, the screams came from someone *other* than the patient.

Let us introduce you to Robert Liston, aka "the fastest knife in the West End."

Liston was a larger-than-life character, half-surgeon and half-entertainer within the operating theater of 1840s Scotland. His amputation surgeries were well attended by students peering over the galleries. Liston, occasionally with knife clasped in teeth, barked at the onlookers, "Time me, gentlemen, time me!"

Time him they did. Liston was fast (his amputations generally took less than three minutes from first cut to wound closure). His speed was so mighty that once he accidentally sliced off the testicles of the patient. A free castration, to boot! Another time, he accidentally cut off the fingers of his assistant (who often held the leg in place); during the procedure, one of the onlookers dropped dead from terror when the knife slashed close enough to cut his coat. Unfortunately, the patient died. The poor assistant also later died of gangrene from the finger amputations, and thus Liston became the proud surgeon who could now boast a stunning 300 *percent* mortality rate from one surgery.

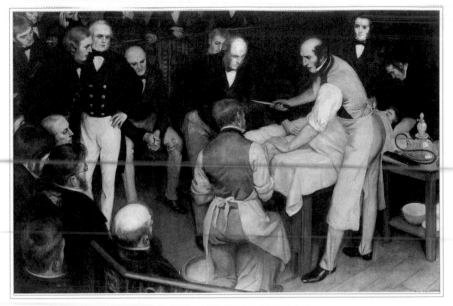

Robert Liston in the operating theater.

The atmosphere surrounding Liston's flamboyant surgeries was not unique; with the advent of modern surgery, audiences were flocking to see these rock stars in action. London and Paris also boasted surgeries that were more akin to Broadway shows. There were ticket sales, with high fees for the most entertaining surgeons, tens to hundreds of spectators, and preoperative celebrity performances. The surgeon was met with applause before and during the procedure. Honoré de Balzac, a contemporary, commented that "the glory of surgeons is like that of actors." This flavor of showboating is unimaginable today, although the idea of the celebrity physician certainly isn't.

PRIDE OF PUS

Everyone likely has glimpsed a modern-day operating room in real life or on TV—painstakingly sterile and shining, with sharp equipment, as well as masks and gloves intended to be used only once and then incinerated.

Operating theaters of the nineteenth century were gross, and people *preferred* them that way.

In the early to mid-1800s, you'd see a table almost blackened from blood and pus from countless preceding surgeries. No surgical gloves were worn— they had yet to be invented. Instruments were often rinsed only in water, if at all, and surgeons' hands mostly went unwashed. And the coat worn by the doctor? It was often so caked in layers of blood that it was stiff—a sign of a "good surgeon."

Even surgeons themselves were not exempt from the dangers that lurked at hospitals and medical schools. Professor Jakob Kolletschka died in 1847 from sepsis after he cut one of his own fingers during an autopsy. Medical students at the Vienna General Hospital in 1840 would bring their unwashed hands directly from autopsies to the obstetrics ward, killing one out of three mothers from childbed fever. In contrast, the ward manned by midwifery pupils had a 3 percent mortality rate. When the students switched wards, the horrible death rates followed the medical students and their bacteria-laden hands. The physician Ignaz Semmelweis, observing this, had the staff do something simple but miraculous: wash their hands with soap and a chlorine solution. Voilà—death rates plummeted. But tragically, no one listened.

In the nineteenth century, Joseph Lister built upon microbiologist Louis Pasteur's germ theory of disease and eventually revolutionized surgery by introducing the concept of antisepsis. Many poo-pooed the idea of bacteria. An Edinburgh professor snorted, "Where are these little beasts . . . has anyone seen them yet?" Another surgeon insisted that "there is good reason to believe that the theory of M. Pasteur, upon which Lister bases his treatment, is unsound." But Lister's theories and the facts—there were fewer deaths when antiseptic chemicals such as carbolic acid and general aseptic cleanliness were used—eventually won out by the turn of the twentieth century. They even named a mouthwash after him: Listerine. And now many of us swish and spit in his honor.

A LITHOTOMY TO REMEMBER

Bransby Cooper was the nephew of the more famous and well-respected surgeon Sir Astley Cooper. The nephew was not a good surgeon, but apparently his uncle insisted on his appointment at Guy's Hospital in London.

The procedure was a simple bladder stone removal, called a lithotomy. Normally, they could be done in about five minutes. Normally, the poor patient was tied up with his knees trussed with a cloth behind his neck, genitals all abloom (hence, the modern use of the lithotomy position, by which women give birth in hospitals). Normally, the surgeon cut between the anus and the scrotal sac (an area called the perineum), into the bladder, fished out the stone, and stitched everything up while the patient screamed bloody hell.

That's not exactly what happened when Bransby Cooper attempted the procedure. He couldn't find the bladder. Then he couldn't find the stone. Every surgical instrument at hand was used before Cooper wormed around with his fingers, trying to fish it out.

The patient by then yelled, "Oh! Let it go! Pray, let it keep in!" But to no avail. Cooper blamed the patient for having a deep perineum before yelping out at the assistant, "Dodd, have you a long finger?" He eventually found the stone, but after a whopping fifty-five minutes. The next day, the patient died, no doubt with a crater-sized hole in his nether region.

After the creator of *The Lancet*, Thomas Wakley, exposed Cooper's incompetency publicly, the doctor sued him for £2000. He ended up winning, but only a trifling £100.

It would turn out to be the first malpractice trial in history—but certainly not the last.

A lithotomy in progress, 1768.

Unfortunately for our twentieth president, James Garfield, his doctors weren't as impressed by Lister. After suffering a nonlethal bullet wound, Garfield was examined by doctors who probed the area with unwashed fingers and instruments. Pus began to form in the wound while he attempted to recover, and the doctors probed yet again with unwashed hands. He died months later, in 1881, due to complications of infection.

Soon, even the public operating theaters and their filthy surfaces disappeared. Cleanliness, hand washing, and surgical gloves became de rigueur. Surgery would no longer be a last resort, but a keenly wielded tactical maneuver in the fight against illness.

First, Do No Harm . . . Oh, Never Mind

Some surgical innovations were skin-crawling but brilliant. In the *Samhita*, written by Indian surgeon Sushruta in 500 BCE, he recommended, "Large black ants should be applied to the margins of the wound and their bodies then severed from their heads, after these have firmly bitten the part with their jaws." Voilá. Insect's mandibles as natural staples for wound closure. Genius, right?

But many surgical history books tell of the not-so-ingenious stories of surgically altering what probably shouldn't be altered. Stuttering is a classic example. In the nineteenth century, German surgeon Johann Friedrich Dieffenbach would cut out a triangular wedge near the root of the tongue to cure stuttering. Others tried to "resize" the tongue, or cut the frenulum, the delicate piece of tissue between the tongue and the floor of the mouth. None of these procedures worked.

In 1831, a Mr. Preston decided that it would be a good idea to tie off a carotid artery on the side where a patient had a stroke. There's just one problem: Strokes often occur from lack of blood flow to the brain. Trying to help by cutting off the blood supply is like helping a drought by telling a rain cloud to do business elsewhere. The patient somehow survived. Preston also recommended that perhaps *both carotid arteries be tied off* for treatment of strokes, epilepsy, and insanity. Thankfully, no one took his advice.

As the fear of autointoxication—the theory that the normal end products of digestion contain poison (see Enemas & Clysters, page 163)—grew, many tried to cure constipation with myriad devices and purgatives at the turn of the twentieth century. One British surgeon, Sir William Arbuthnot Lane, took it a step further. He cut out the colon altogether. He performed more than a thousand colectomies, mostly on women. Surely, slow colons were the cause of women's mental shortcomings like stupidity, headaches,

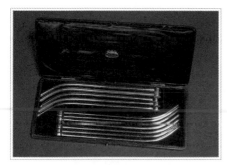

Urethral probes, circa 1870.

and irritability. Luckily, you can snip out your colon and survive, but you'll likely have the side effect of lots of diarrhea. Like most functioning parts of your body, colons are better left intact.

Lane also was a proponent of fixing misplaced organs. Yes, you heard that correctly. In the early twentieth century, many believed that vague abdominal and whole-body discomfort could be due to "dropped" or "misplaced" organs. The kidney was perhaps the most misplaced organ of all time. Lane blamed dropped kidneys, or nephroptosis, for causing suicidality, homicidality, depression, abdominal pain, headaches, and the more obvious physical symptoms of urinary problems. Removing even one kidney killed too many patients, so surgeons instead performed a "nephropexy"—more or less tacking kidneys back in place using sutures and occasionally rubber bands and wads of gauze. By the 1920s, this procedure was falling out of favor with some surgeons claiming that "the most serious complication of nephroptosis is nephropexy" and that urologists seemed to have "an orgy of fixation of kidneys." (To be fair, part of a urologist's job is to fixate on kidneys, but the orgy part was a bit dramatic.)

Kidneys weren't the only body part atrociously fiddled with by surgeons. Tonsils, the glands at the back of the throat, were also removed in excessive numbers in an effort to put a stop to all childhood infections—a well-meaning but misguided aim. Of course, the tonsillectomy has its place as a modern-day therapeutic in cases of sleep apnea and recurrent tonsillitis, but as a last resort. Most would be shocked that in 1934, a study in New York showed that of one thousand children, more than six hundred of them had had tonsillectomies. They weren't risk-free surgeries, either; many children died annually from the procedure. The promise of post-op ice cream was so not worth that.

And no discussion of unnecessary surgery would be complete without a story of pointless fiddling with men's tender nether regions. John Harvey Kellogg, health practitioner and cereal inventor, recommended circumcision to quell evil urges to masturbate if other methods—including bandaging genitals, covering them with cages, and tying hands—failed. The procedure should be done "without administering an anaesthetic, as the brief pain attending the operation will have a salutary effect upon the mind, especially if it be connected with the idea of punishment." Yow. Well, as any circumcised man can tell you, the procedure doesn't prevent masturbation.

THE LURE OF THE SCALPEL CONTINUES

The public has always been lured by the promise of a quick slash and cut to fix everything. Some people love being patients so much they'll go under the knife for fake symptoms, while others repeatedly return to the OR in search of a phantomlike physical perfection. But unlike in past centuries, surgeons and hospitals are under rigorous scrutiny for cleanliness, quality training, low mortality rates, and results that stand both the test of time and the scientific magnifying lens. And thanks to the development of anesthesia, we no longer require the hastiness of the two-minute slash and saw. Thank goodness for that.

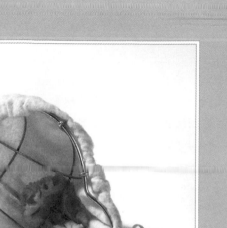

18

Anesthesia

Of Suffocation, Soporific Sponges, Chloroform, Laughing Gas, Doping the Pets, Ether Frolics, and Noxious Farting

Conquering pain is no easy feat. *Anesthesia,* from the Greek words for "absence of sensation," has been sought after since humankind first dared to drill a hole in a head for surgery. Ancient China used hashish. The Egyptians turned to opium. Dioscorides recommended deadly mandrake with wine. In the Middle Ages, there were even recipes for a "soporific sponge," soaked in mandrake, henbane, hemlock, and opium, then dried in the sun. It was then rinsed in hot water, squeezed but left damp, and applied to the patient's nose for inhalation.

The problem with using alcohol or other substances like it is that you need a lot—as in poisonous quantities—to prevent someone from waking during surgery. So other methods were developed. Stories are told of men being whacked in the head for a concussion-induced sleep before castration in ancient China. Obviously, we had a ways to go.

It took a lot of trial, error, and more than a few doped pets to reach our modern era of painless medical procedures. Several chapters in the annals of anesthesia were written by some hard-partying, borderline sociopathic characters. So the next time you blissfully awaken from a surgery, remember to thank the child-stranglers, sponge-huffers, and ether frolickers of the past. Let us introduce you to a few of them.

Carbon Dioxide Gonna Knock You Out

Henry Hill Hickman was a puppy killer. One of the fathers of modern anesthesia, the British physician tested his theories of "suspended animation" on animals in the early nineteenth century. He used carbonic acid gas (what is now known as carbon dioxide) as an inhalant thusly:

> I took a puppy a month old . . . and placed a glass cover so as to prevent the access of atmospheric air; in ten minutes, he showed great marks of uneasiness, in 12 respiration became difficult, and in 17 minutes ceased altogether, at 18 minutes I took off one of the Ears . . . and the animal did not appear to be the least sensible of pain.

Let us pause for a moment to weep for the test subject.
Oh, for crying out loud, that poor puppy!
So yes, Hickman was suffocating puppies—sometimes to death. But he wasn't the first to use asphyxiation as anesthesia: Some claim that the Assyrians used to strangle children into unconsciousness to perform circumcisions—also a practice in Italy until the seventeenth century.

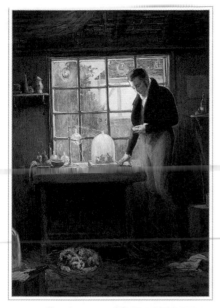

Henry Hill Hickman. Note the unconscious or possibly dead puppy under the glass.

(Strangulation before genital cutting? No, no, no. Hell no.) And the truth was, it worked! When you're deeply unconscious from lack of oxygen, you too can have your ear or your nether regions painlessly chopped off.

But the problem was, it killed, too. Hickman smartly included only the positive results when he reported his methods. But the medical community saw through the charade: He was either ignored or given scathing reviews. This one from *The Lancet*, entitled "Surgical Humbug," said that the world would "laugh him to scorn if he were to recommend a man who was about to have a tooth drawn to be previously hanged, drowned, or smothered for a few minutes, in order that he may feel no pain during the operation." The writer also called Hickman's work a "tissue of Quackery" and "humbug" and signed this piece of work, "I am, &tc, ANTIQUACK."

Ouch. One wonders if Hickman gave himself a dose of carbon dioxide to render himself senseless after that burn. Still, it's a good thing that Hickman's idea didn't take off. After all, carbon dioxide as an anesthetic is as good as using a noose. Fatal suffocation is an irreversible side effect.

CHLOROFORM: INHALE DEEPLY . . .

Edinburgh physician James Young Simpson was another nineteenth-century pioneer in anesthesia. That is, if pioneering meant inhaling random substances with your colleagues, just to see what would happen. After

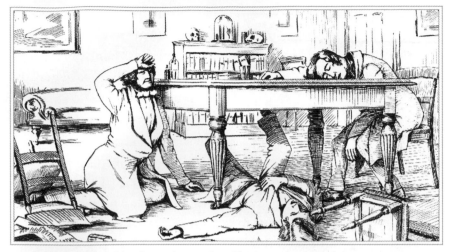

James Young Simpson and friends meet their match in chloroform.

fishing a bottle of chloroform from under a pile of trash (he had assumed it was probably not worth the try before), he and his friends started sniffing deeply. Chloroform has a sickly sweet smell, and before long giddiness sets in with a buzzing in the ears and heavy limbs. The inhalers began laughing (the "preliminary stage of excitement," Simpson explained), then talking way too much, before *bam!* They all fell unconscious, and in the process, trashed the dining room where the sniffing occurred.

After they awoke, they decided chloroform was pretty awesome, so they sniffed it multiple times to make sure it rendered them as silly and unconscious as it had before. Mrs. Simpson's niece joined in, exclaiming, "I'm an angel! Oh, I'm an angel!" before passing out.

Chloroform is a simple molecule. Take methane (the main component of natural gas), replace three of its hydrogens with three chlorines, and you get chloroform. Simpson soon began championing chloroform as anesthesia in surgery, and it became an attraction during the mid-nineteenth-century party frolics that also featured ether sniffing (more on that later).

As with most drugs that mask pain, it wasn't long before we started confusing comfort with cure. Perhaps people figured, *If it makes me feel woozy and numb, surely it's good for me.* Chloroform began showing up in various pharmaceuticals, like Gibson's Linseed Licorice and Chloroform Lozenges and Bee Brand White Pine and Tar Cough Syrup. They claimed to help all diseases of the throat and lungs (though chloroform is actually quite irritating) and to cure tuberculosis (they didn't). Other nostrums promised to help ills such as vomiting, diarrhea, insomnia, and pain. As a sedative, it made sense for those latter complaints, but chloroform is far from a perfect cure-all. It's deadly.

"Sudden sniffer's death" killed one too many patients given chloroform. Healthy patients died inexplicably, due to heart arrhythmias, as well as respiratory and heart failure. Chloroform can also cause liver and kidney toxicity and is probably carcinogenic. By the twentieth century, it fell out of favor due to its dangers and is now a remnant of murder mysteries as a favorite (albeit imperfect) killing agent.

Rolling on the Floor Laughing My Gas Off

Apparently, finding new gases for people to inhale was all the rage in the United Kingdom in the eighteenth century. The Pneumatic Institution for Relieving Diseases by Medical Airs opened in the late 1700s in Bristol, and its founders tried a lot of dubious treatments. Humphry Davy, who joined in 1798 and contributed breakthroughs on respiratory physiology and anesthesia, had a scary method to figure out whether certain gases were safe or not: He inhaled them himself. (Are you sensing a pattern with anesthesia pioneers?)

Carbon monoxide was one such gas. He noted: "I seemed to be sinking into annihilation" but luckily didn't die. With hydrogen gas: "A bystander informed me that . . . my cheeks became purple." Brave dude. But he did realize that nitrous oxide, also known as laughing gas, took away toothache pain in 1800. He also realized it could make you nauseous, after he thoughtfully

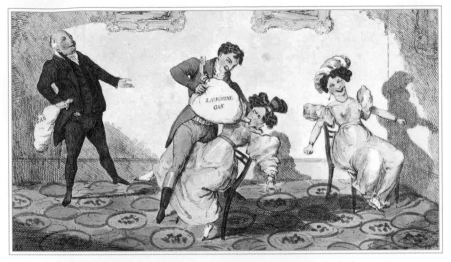

The original title of this piece was "Prescription for Scolding Wives." Women's rights had a ways to go.

drank a bottle of wine in eight minutes flat, took a five-quart hit of laughing gas, and immediately puked.

Oh, and the Pneumatic Institution? It closed after none of the gases they experimented with actually cured lung diseases, including tuberculosis. Davy's research was forgotten for some time, partly because of the Pneumatic Institution's complete failure to heal anyone and partly because Davy switched his curious mind from soporific subjects to a more energizing field of study—electrophysiology.

Nitrous oxide for medicinal purposes was shelved for the time being. But it would become a recreational drug used at parties for several decades in the nineteenth century. It wasn't until 1844 that American dentist Horace Wells decided to continue investigating Davy's previously unacknowledged anesthetic properties of the gas. Wells had his own tooth pulled under nitrous oxide and, finding it painless, went public. He built a breathing apparatus and asked surgeon John Collins Warren (a founder of Massachusetts General Hospital and the *New England Journal of Medicine and Surgery*) to perform an amputation using the gas. When the patient refused, a volunteer medical student from the crowd

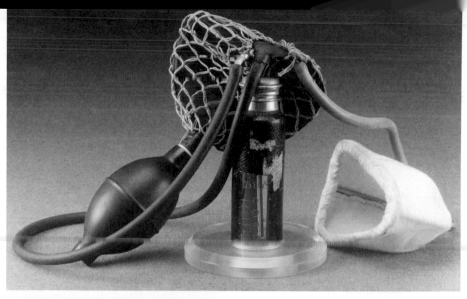

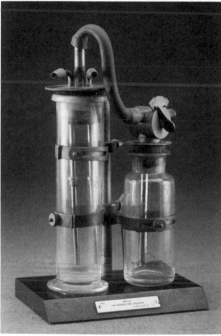

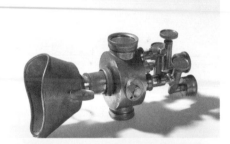

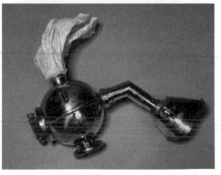

Clockwise, from lower left: Boyle's apparatus, which allowed for greater control over the flow of anesthesia (1917); the Junker inhaler, first to use a rubber bellows to move air over the liquid (1867); anesthesia face mask (early 1900s); the Ombredanne inhaler, with a felt-packed metal sphere for absorbing liquid ether (1907); another face mask, with bottles of chloroform.

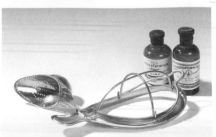

allowed a tooth to be extracted. The gas wasn't given properly—perhaps Wells's new apparatus failed—and the student felt everything.

Poor Wells suffered horrible embarrassment and would eventually become addicted to chloroform. He grew mentally unstable and, after throwing sulfuric acid onto prostitutes, committed suicide in the infamous Tombs prison in New York City.

Later in the 1860s, dentists gave nitrous oxide another chance. Other medical professionals adopted it in lieu of ether and chloroform, both of which were problematic. Perhaps Wells sleeps more soundly in his grave knowing that nitrous oxide continues to be used as a sedative to this day.

Perhaps not.

NO HUMBUG? LET'S FROLIC!

William Morton was a Boston dentist who'd attended the failed demonstration of Horace Wells. Morton wouldn't make the same mistake. Instead of nitrous oxide, he investigated ether inhalation. "Sweet oil of vitriol," also known as diethyl ether, ethyl ether, or just plain ether, was first synthesized in the sixteenth century by adding sulfuric acid to ethanol. It was used (uselessly) for treatment of respiratory infections, bladder stones, and scurvy in the eighteenth century. But in the 1840s, its use as an anesthetic had finally arrived.

Morton placed drops of it on the gums of his patients before tooth extractions and found it anesthetized the area. The next step? He started dousing his pet goldfish with it. His wife, Elizabeth, wasn't happy about this, but Morton continued. He began eyeing their pet spaniel, Nig. Elizabeth put her foot down, but Morton anesthetized little Nig anyway. One can imagine that marriage wasn't exactly blissful in the Morton household.

On October 16, 1846, Morton took his findings to a public exhibition with the same Dr. Warren who'd performed the botched procedure with Wells and nitrous oxide. In a surgical theater at Massachusetts General Hospital,

Warren removed a neck tumor from a patient under ether anesthesia, directed by Morton. At the close of surgery, as the patient woke up, pain-free, Dr. Warren announced, "Gentlemen, this is no humbug!"

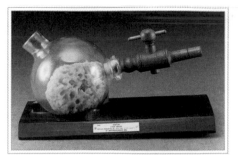

A replica of Morton's ether inhaler.

(The definition of *humbug*, we should have mentioned, is deceptive or false behaviors. It is also a peppermint candy, but surely Dr. Warren meant the former.)

The surgical theater at Mass General was soon nicknamed "The Ether Dome" (not a Mad Max movie) and the historical date, Ether Day. Unfortunately, Morton took his discovery down an exploitative and quackish road. He colored the ether and put in additives to mask the scent, renaming it "Letheon" after the mythical Greek river, Lethe, which imparted oblivion and forgetfulness to drinkers. He patented Letheon a month after that fateful

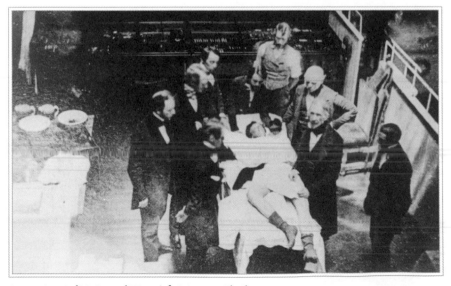

A reenactment of Morton and Warren's first surgery with ether.

introduction to the world, though it was soon obvious his patent was simply for ether. The medical community in America and abroad derided Morton for trying to keep the discovery—an easily created substance—from benefitting mankind. Morton's reputation never recovered.

But ether's reputation continued to gain ground. Shortly after Morton's initial successful demonstration, Oliver Wendell Holmes coined the term *anesthesia* in a private letter to him. Ether was soon used extensively for surgical anesthesia, which is great, except for three problems—it was highly flammable, caused nausea and vomiting, and irritated the lungs (which is interesting, given that physicians used it to treat pulmonary inflammation a century earlier). Also, it had a really stinky odor that stuck with patients.

It had developed another reputation—one for recreational abuse and quack medicines.

Ether showed up on shelves to treat colic and diarrhea. Hoffman's Drops, containing one part ether to three parts alcohol, was said to cure feminine ills such as cramps but easily became an addictive cure-all.

What was worse, ether abuse was socially acceptable. In the mid-nineteenth century, parties called ether frolics or jags became common. Participants would inhale ether, making them giddy, intoxicated, and often unconscious. One of the physicians who participated, Crawford Long, was a slimeball about it. After getting a supply, he boasted, "We have some girls in Jefferson who are anxious to see it taken, and you know nothing would afford me more pleasure than to take it in their presence and to get a few sweet kisses." What a lech.

It wasn't all frolicking about with gross men. Recreational users would wake up with bruises and injuries. Some died. One gentleman unfortunately smoked tobacco while using ether, and an onlooker noted, "Won day after a dose uv it, he wint to light his pipe and the fire cot his breath and tuk fire inside."

One physician, a Dr. Kelly in Ireland, decided that ether would be the cure for alcoholism. Sure, just switch one addictive substance for another; that'll do. "Dr. Kelly's Remedy" was given to patients as a nonalcoholic alternative. It was a "liquor on which a man could get drunk with a clean conscience." Sure it was. But many towns began to reek from the ether stink, literally (it smells pungent, sweet, but with an unpleasant solvent odor). Finally, the British government classified ether as a poison and began to regulate its sale in 1891.

Good thing, too. Besides being addictive, flammable, and occasionally deadly, ether caused some pretty profound burping, hiccuping, and noxious farting.

ANESTHETICS TODAY

Today, most of us will have used anesthetics at some point in our lives, whether it be for a tooth pulling or surgery. We owe a lot to the horrible experimentation and occasional unhappy endings that accompany these histories. Chloroform and ether anesthetics have been culled from the shelves and hospitals, as safer medicines, including sedative-hypnotic agents such as propofol (nicknamed "milk of amnesia" for its white color), opioids such as fentanyl, benzodiazepines such as midazolam, and many others have replaced them. We have become ever more specific in how anesthetics are used. Local nerve-blocking drugs such as novocaine make dental procedures painless. Spinal and epidural anesthesia minimize side effects like breathing problems or cardiac risks from general anesthesia. Though extremely safe these days, general anesthesia inherently carries with it drug-specific risks, including death—which increases the sicker you are going into surgery.

Lulling the human body into a short-term comatose state with a Lazarus happy ending is not to be done carelessly or with just any drug. And for the record, it's a good thing that laughing gas/chloroform/ether parties are over. People would have to find other legal (or illegal) ways to frolic instead.

The Men's Health Hall of Shame

The *Oxford English Dictionary* defines *virile* as "having strength, energy, and a strong sexual drive." Merriam-Webster cuts to the chase, defining *virility* simply as "manhood." We can thank ancient Greece and Rome, where brawniness was combined with self-control, confidence, political engagement, sexual proliferation, and high levels of energy to create a masculine ideal that—with some variations—has been passed down to us through the ages.

Now, of course, achieving the masculine ideal of virility is fraught with complications and the potential for insecurities. Men everywhere are plagued with nagging questions of self-doubt: What if I lose this competition? What if I don't get this job? What if I can't grow a beard? What if I go bald? What if I can't "get it up"?

These are the thoughts that have kept men awake at night throughout the history of Western civilization. And these fears have always been exploited for financial gain by quack medical practitioners. Exhibit A: An advertisement for the "perfect male organ developer" (an early vacuum device for erectile dysfunction) boldly stated that "A man who is sexually weak is unfit to marry. Weak men hate themselves." What follows are a few quack-endorsed ways for weak men to hate themselves a little less.

NUXATED IRON

What do baseball great Ty Cobb, boxing champion Jack Dempsey, and Pope Benedict XV all have in common? All three offered high-profile endorsements to "Nuxated Iron." Latching on

to the eternal male quests for vitality and virility, "Nuxated Iron" claimed to restore "bodily or mental vigor" by increasing iron levels in your bloodstream. Although the product did indeed contain ferrous sulfate (iron) and a tasty touch of oil of cinnamon, it also contained nux vomica (strychnine), a neurotoxin that would, if taken in a high enough dose, poison you. Horrifically. (See Strychnine, page 72.)

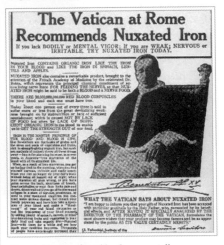

Nuxated Iron endorsed by the pope, y'all.

THE STEPHENSON SPERMATIC TRUSS

The Stephenson Spermatic Truss arrived on the scene in 1876, ready to help curb men of their masturbatory tendencies by providing a cumbersome and inconvenient way to tie your penis to your leg. Apparently the device wasn't quite effective enough, as later versions included little spikes that would bite into your penis should you have the misfortune of becoming aroused.

THE STRINGER SELF-TREATING DEVICE

The dubiously named Stringer self-treating device combined every possible method of keeping the penis erect into one package. The company promoted it as "four in one—vacuum, moist-heat, vibration, and electricity." And the device managed to combine hot water, an induction coil, an electric current, a vacuum, and even an electrode that could be coated with Vaseline and inserted a few inches into the rectum for the added benefit of a "prostate massage." The company assured consumers that it "was the most wonderful discovery since the world began."

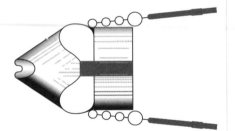

The Bowen Device in all its terrible glory.

THE BOWEN DEVICE

Intended to discourage masturbation, the Bowen would not seem out of place in the sex toy chest of a dominatrix today. It was basically a penis cap attached to the pubic hair by little chains. The more aroused you got, the more the little chains pulled on your pubic hair. Ouch.

THE FIRST PENIS RING

Around 1200 the first penis rings were invented in China. Creatively made from, of all things, the eyelids of a goat, the penis rings purposefully left the eyelashes intact to increase sexual pleasure. Let that visual sink in for a moment. A few hundred years later, the Chinese moved on to ivory rings, an obvious improvement for both men and goats.

THE PROSTATE GLAND WARMER

The Electro Thermal Company of Ohio manufactured a rectal gland warmer called the Thermalaid, which ran an electric current, regulated by a light bulb, through its hard rubber exterior in an effort to "stimulate the abdominal brain."

"If a rectal dilator is used it will furnish a constant heat to the rectal anatomy, causing a gentle stimulation of the capillary blood vessels and the resultant improved local nerve condition."

The regulatory light bulb inevitably led to some awkward encounters. "Hi honey, I'm home, saw you had a light on late and—oh my God, what are you doing?"

THE RECTO ROTOR

This vicious-looking device was inserted into the rectum, where it would lubricate the prostate and colon and "massage the muscles of the rectal region." The advertisements assured consumers that they could be used by the patient himself "in the privacy of his own home," thus sparing the user the embarrassment of using a Recto Rotor in public. The size of the rotor was also advertised as "large enough to be efficient, small enough for anyone more than fifteen years old." And that just raises all sorts of troubling questions, doesn't it?

SPRAY-ON HAIR

If you had a sleepover sometime in the 1990s, you probably caught an infomercial late at night where baldness and thinning hair were hidden by an aerosol can of "spray-on hair." The product, called GLH (short for "Great Looking Hair"), was as ridiculous as it sounds (only $39.92!), but the infomercial is worth tracking down on YouTube for the testimonial of a deeply unfortunate young man with both a mullet and a receding hairline, who boldly claims that after using GLH "the babes are back." Spray-on hair still has a market today. Thanks, mullet man.

MUSCLE STIMULATORS

Looking to tone your muscles without actually doing anything? Electronic muscle stimulator (EMS) machines "work" the muscles by jolting them with electricity, causing involuntary contractions. The Executive Briefcase model from Executive Fitness Products, however, also caused another involuntary reaction: cardiac arrhythmias. The FDA ordered the destruction of the machines in 1996.

BEARD GENERATORS

Probably the worst time in history to be alive as a man who couldn't grow facial hair was Victorian England (or Portland, Oregon, in the noughties) when chest-length beards, bushy sideburns, and elaborate mustaches were all the rage.

To help, an advertisement for a topical treatment called Professor Modevi's Beard Generator ran in London newspapers, claiming to generate robust beard growth from a scant four to six weeks of use, even by "young men not above seventeen years of age." [Ingredients not stated.]

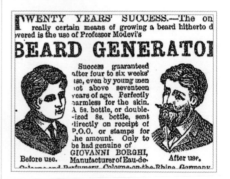

Watch a boy become a man before your very eyes.

ANIMALS

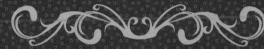

Creepy Crawlies, Corpses,
and the Healing Power of the Human Body

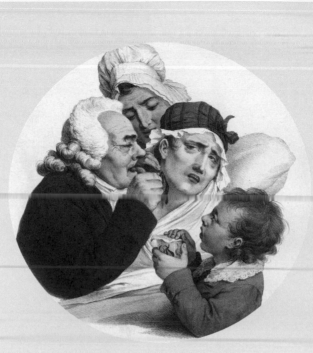

19

Leeches

Of Leech Pendants, Mercedes-Benz Bites, Leech Fight Club, Drunken Cannibal Worms, and the Predicament of Asslessness

In 1850 London, a physician makes a house call on a woman with a nagging sore throat. Clearly, swollen tonsils are to blame. Clearly, decongesting and shrinking them will solve the problem. Clearly, the answer to the problem is . . . leeches.

From a portable earthenware jar, he withdraws a single dark, slimy, squirming leech, about three inches long. It wriggles briskly from hunger. He pierces the tail end with silk-threaded needle, then pushes the writhing leech "pendant" into a clear glass tube, to direct the leech's hungry mouth onto the offending tonsil. The leech sinks its tiny, toothy jaws onto the swollen tissue, but the patient hardly feels the bite. After all, the leech's best offense is to be as inoffensive as possible. Stealth biting is a good thing.

There is a ticklish sensation from the squirming. The leech swells larger and larger, until replete with blood. It detaches happily and is yanked away by its tether. The patient feels a trickle of salty blood at the back of her mouth for an hour or more.

This gag-worthy scene was incredibly commonplace in history. After all, the leech has been sucking blood out of the human race, with our permission, for a long, long time.

THE ORIGINS OF LEECHCRAFT

Leeches and bloodletting were believed to accomplish the same goal—relieving the body "congested" of blood and inflammation. By bleeding away the "bad" blood, you could potentially bleed away the problem. *Any problem.* The reasons for leeching were many, including venereal diseases, brain inflammation, epilepsy, hysteria, organ disease, and tuberculosis.

So who's responsible for bringing leeches into our lives? You can start with the Egyptians, whose tombs document the earliest use of leeching, for curing fever-borne illnesses and flatulence, as far back as 1500 BCE. In Homer's *Iliad*, Podalirius, one of the sons of Asclepius, was a healer and referred to as a *leech*. Then there's the ancient Chinese story claiming leech therapy began when King Hui (d. 430 BCE) accidentally swallowed one in his salad and was surprised to find that his stomach ailments improved.

Nineteenth-century leech jar.

But leeching *really* took off with the theories of Hippocrates in the fourth century BCE and, later, Galen in the second century CE. Both physicians firmly established the idea that bleeding could bring balance to the humors. These distinct bodily elements, considered to be the source of health and disease, drove the theories of Western medical care for nearly two centuries.

After Hippocrates and Galen, we begin to see more and more evidence of leech use for everything from removing evil spirits (Themison of Laodicea, Syria) to treating hearing loss (Alexander de Tralles). One medieval physician even claimed that it "sharpens the hearing, stops tears, . . . and produces a musical voice." If only we could all just apply a squirmy bloodsucker and become Beyoncé.

So if leeching and bloodletting accomplish the same goal, why use a slimy creature instead of a lancet to let the blood flow?

LEECH VS. LANCET

First, consider the animal itself. *Hirudo medicinalis*, the lofty Latin name for the common medical leech, was born to suck blood. For starters, its saliva contains a blood thinner (hirudin) that keeps blood from clotting and ensures an ample flow. And to digest the meal? These creatures put mammals and their one or two or three stomachs to shame by having ten stomachs for digesting. The leech is also overachieving teeth-wise. It has three jaws, with about one hundred teeth per jaw. That's a three-hundred-tooth bite, which leaves behind a mark in the shape of the Mercedes Benz hood ornament.

Unlike lancets, fleams, or bladed scarificators, a leech bite was relatively painless, thanks to its saliva. A genius concoction of chemicals, leech spit thoughtfully contains anesthetics to keep its host comfy and unaware, useful in the wild when an irritating scratch from a host could end a feeding before it started. The ancient Sanskrit text *Sushruta Samhita*, which discussed the use of leeches instead of regular bloodletting on "imbeciles" and "persons of extreme timid disposition," praised the practice as a "gentler" therapy.

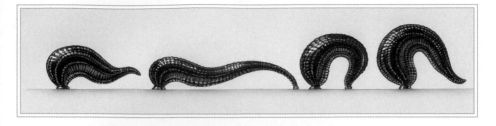

Leeches also allowed for more accurate, targeted bleeding. Bloodletting was often done on the upper arms, but in smaller, tighter areas, something smaller and tidier was needed. Because leeching practitioners thought that the bloodletting ought to occur closest to the area of problem, the bloodsuckers were placed on the temples for headaches, behind the ears for vertigo, on the back of the head for lethargy, on the belly for stomach ailments, and over the spleen for epilepsy. And for menstrual afflictions, they'd be placed on the upper thighs, vulva, and sometimes directly on the cervix. In fact, leeching chairs were created with holes in the seat area to apply anal leeches.

A leech has three jaws, 300 teeth, and a distinct Mercedes logo–shaped bite.

Commence uncomfortable leg crossing right about *now*.

Oh, don't worry! It gets worse, which brings us to our next point: Leeches could go where lancets couldn't—*inside the body*. Sometimes, a good anal bleeding wasn't enough. Internal management was necessary, especially for intestinal inflammation and prostate problems. There was just one snag: The worms would be, ahem, forcefully ejected. One clever physician created a grooved metal rod designed for holding and inserting threaded leeches to good effect. It was quite fancy, with a nice leather handle. In 1833, a Dr. Osborne described the procedure. After shoving the leeches deep into the anus, "The instrument

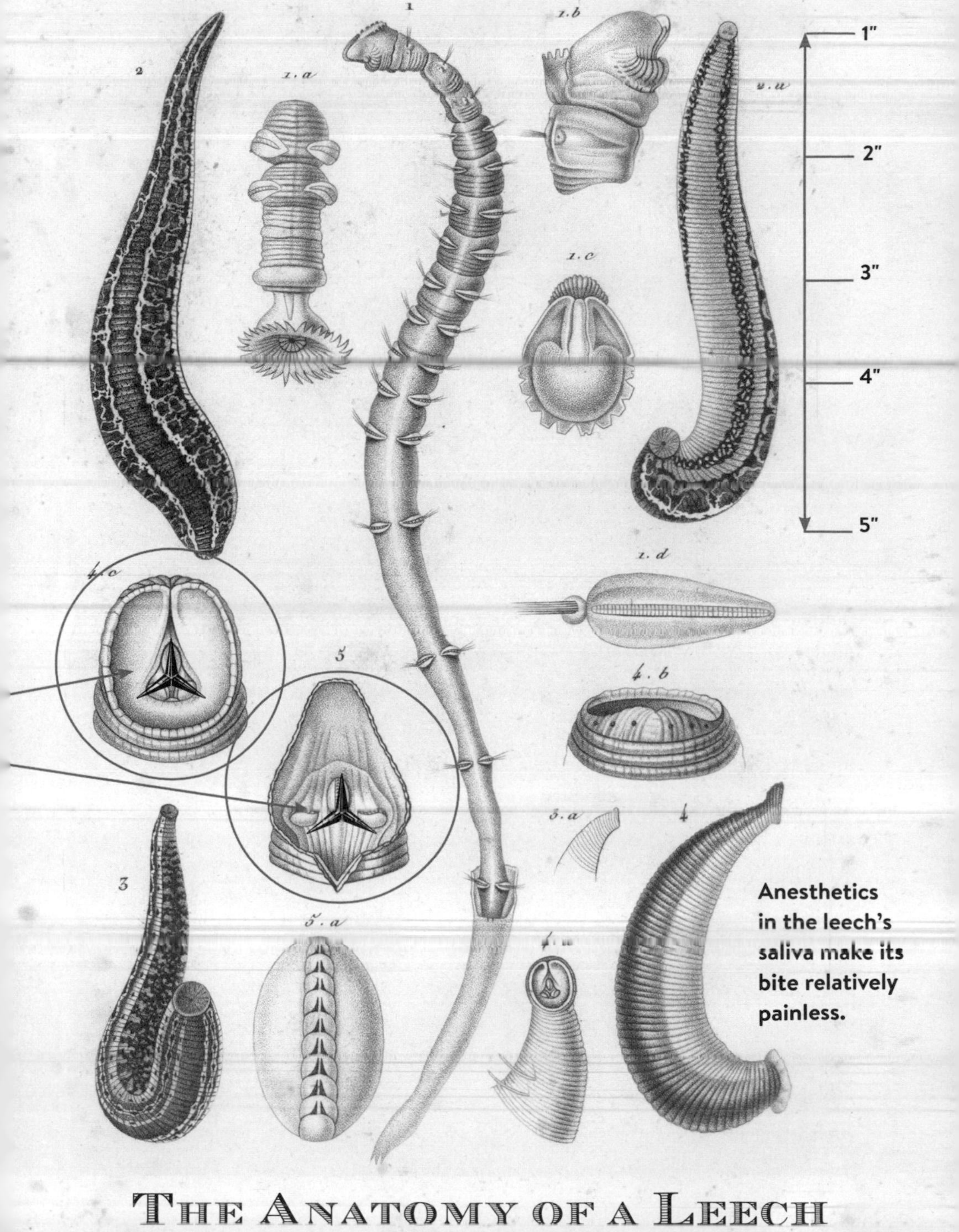

1"
2"
3"
4"
5"

Anesthetics
in the leech's
saliva make its
bite relatively
painless.

THE ANATOMY OF A LEECH

is withdrawn, and the leeches are suffered to remain till gorged with blood." It seems that "suffered" is the apt word in this scenario. Poor things. Poor person.

Leeches were also used in the vagina to either stimulate menstrual flow or treat painful menses, but it was noted that this particular use should be "confined to married women" and "a clever nurse should be taught to apply them." We sincerely hope she was paid well for this.

MAKING THE MOST OF YOUR LEECH

As for prime leeching conditions, leeches prefer to bite clean, freshly shaved skin. No stubble! "I have found the sharp points of the incised hairs so greatly to annoy them," declared Mr. Wilkinson, a leech expert in 1804 London. Something to remember when wading in muddy ponds—prickly legs can be a good thing. But even with the smoothest of skin, the dainty beasts sometimes needed a little coaxing. The Lancet reported in 1848 that they bit more vigorously if dunked in a nice dark beer or some diluted wine. The area of skin could be bathed in milk, sugar water, or best, a little bit of fresh blood. Even a tiny knick from a knife tip could do the trick. This latter technique is still used today.

After fifteen minutes or so, the blood-filled leech usually fell off the patient, but occasionally the practitioner had to remove it. A sprinkling of table salt over the leech's head helped because yanking it off might traumatize the skin. If the leech appeared to have fallen asleep from a food coma, a hard flick of the finger and a splash of water quickly revived it.

Often after leeches were removed, further bleeding was coaxed from the bites by wrapping the area in warm linen to dilate the patient's blood vessels. Others recommended perpetuating the ooze by submerging the patient in a warm bath.

In 1816, Dr. James Rawlins Johnson published his *Treatise on the Medicinal Leech*. Besides the aforementioned methods of leech use, he studied the leech itself with exacting care. He tested to see if they were cannibals (they were); he froze them with or without salt to see if they would die (snow plus salt was worse). He even had leech fights between burly horse leeches and medicinal leeches (the horse leeches won). He also tortured them with carbonic acid, mercury, gas pumps, and olive oil, and was surprised to find that the leech "is very tenacious of life." (The authors stopped reading after they reached this choice sentence: "Hermaphroditic impregnation may occur in a single leech." The visual is . . . never mind. Just don't.)

As noted earlier, leeches were used inside the body, as well as outside. This, of course, begs the question: How to get the parasites out? Philip Crampton, an avid practitioner in 1822, had a solution: Thread the poor things. After applying these leeches directly to swollen tonsils, he noted that threading "causes them to bite with increased ardor, and, in fact, may be used to stimulate torpid leeches."

They needn't have worried: If a leech was swallowed, it would likely be digested by stomach acid. But not knowing this, medieval practitioners recommended gargling with goat urine, coaxing the leech out with a cautery iron, or making the patient thirsty as to "bait" it to crawl out for a refreshing drink of water. The ends did not justify the means by any extent because it didn't work. Come to think of it, *nothing* justifies the drinking of goat urine.

There was also the matter of recycling. Leeches weren't always tossed after a feeding. They could be reused up to fifty times if the animals were "encouraged" to disgorge: just dab a little salt on their mouths (which is really starting to sound like the leech equivalent of dabbing hydrochloric acid on a human). The leeches would then vomit like Ozzy Osbourne in his heyday. The cost savings were considerable. Other doctors would drop the engorged leeches into vinegar (a whole bath of acid!) and they'd perk up. Or so we imagine. In this manner, they could be used twice a week for up to three years.

The care and keeping of leeches was no small task. Mr. Wilkinson explained, "In short, so much patience, as well as dexterity, is required in the management of these capricious, or rather irritable animals."

Sounds like Mr. Wilkinson wanted to bite the leeches right back.

DRAWBACKS AND THE WORMY DOWNFALL

Leeching had its drawbacks. The classic Mercedes-Benz bite sign wasn't exactly a badge of honor. Despite a short time when leeches were fashionable (leech shapes were embroidered onto dresses in the nineteenth century), people often covered their bites in public.

Remember that whole "reuse" thing? Before "single-use leeches" and other medical equipment were introduced, multiuse leeches could create more problems than they fixed. One report in 1827 showed how a leech was used for a syphilitic patient, then reused to treat a child, who then contracted the disease.

Another limitation of the leech was the fact that it could take in only about a tablespoon of blood. To keep a continuous flow, one could snip off the tail and let the ingested blood flow freely. It's a sort of Sisyphean method to leechcraft. They eat and eat, and never get full, and they have become completely assless. And then they die. What a life.

Some patients died from overenthusiastic leeching, as in the case of a two-year-old girl in 1819 who died of a hemorrhage from a single bite. Because of the long-lasting blood-thinning properties in leech spit, patients could continue to bleed well after the leeching. Often, a single treatment was not enough. The numbers could be staggering. François-Joseph-Victor Broussais, one of the most sanguinary of physicians from the nineteenth century, applied up to fifty leeches at a time. Another physician applied 130 leeches to a poor soul's testicle for gonorrhea treatment. It is, perhaps, one of the best advertisements for STD safe-sex campaigns.

If that weren't enough, the bites themselves could become contaminated with dangerous, life-threatening infections. Nineteenth-century medical literature is riddled with case reports in which the bites became the focus of problems.

FRESH LEECHES FOR SALE!

Where did one acquire a leech? At the turn of the nineteenth century, poor English children would wade into murky freshwater and sell the leeches clinging to their legs for pocket money. But soon, leeches became scarce. Even baiting your fish line with chunks of liver did no good.

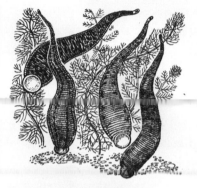

By the 1830s, England's consumption of leeches hit an all-time high. Leeches were being imported from Turkey, India, Egypt, and Australia. Forty-two million leeches were imported to England from France in a single year. The United States loved leeching, too, but its home-grown *Macrobdella decora* had a smaller bite and drew less blood, so they also imported *Hirudo medicinalis*.

Soon, *hirudiculture*, or leech farming, emerged to meet the demand. At these "leecheries," cows, donkeys, and decrepit horses were driven into muddy waters or marshes, sometimes slashed with cuts to encourage feeding. In 1863, the *British Medical Journal* noted, rightly so, that "Hiruduculture is a tolerably disgusting business." Today, leech farming is clean cut, complete with filtered water systems and scientifically organized breeding. Not a poverty-stricken kid or decrepit horse in sight.

Unlike lancets, leeches were high maintenance. They were, after all, finicky eaters and somewhat unpredictable. It's not easy to get a leech to bite exactly where you want it to, and thus custom glass leech tubes were used for application. Special jars were used to carry them around town. So much work!

By the mid-nineteenth century, a growing crowd of physicians began to earnestly denounce "heroic depletion therapy," thanks to a more solid understanding of physiology, pathology, and a certain something called statistics. One of the founding fathers of evidence-based medicine was Pierre Louis, who was a staunch defender of facts over vague theorizing. He found no convincing evidence that bloodletting was efficacious. Others, like John Hughes Bennett, followed suit.

By the early twentieth century, bloodletting and leechcraft for any random illness had, well, bled out.

THE MODERN "BITING EDGE" OF MEDICINE TODAY

Many would be shocked and surprised to hear that leeches are still used for legitimate reasons. (Also, thank goodness for antibiotics. No one really wants a leech sucking on their strep throat, right?)

For one thing, there was the discovery of hirudin by John Berry Haycraft in 1884. Hirudin is the main blood-thinning protein in leech saliva. Now, milking itty-bitty leeches for their oral secretions, rattlesnake-style, isn't really possible. So scientists instead synthesized versions of hirudin, and still use them today as clot-busting and clot-preventing anticoagulants.

The leech's ability to bite small areas of the body, remove unwanted blood, and prevent blood clotting are beneficial in the right situation. After reconstructive surgeries for delicate, small areas such as fingers, ears, and nose tips, leeches can gently decompress tissues engorged with blood, and by doing so, improve blood flow and the survival rate of those tissues. In free flap reconstructions, where whole sections of flesh and skin, together with their blood vessels and nerves, are sewn onto new areas (such as head and neck reconstructions after a life-saving cancer removal), leeches have prevented swollen tissues from cutting off delicate blood supply.

So in some cases, leeches are good for you! It almost makes you want to snuggle up with a slimy critter to say thank you.

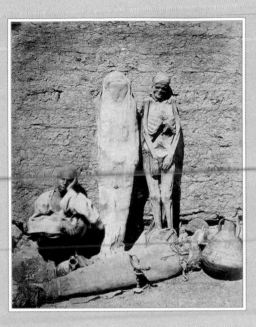

20

Cannibalism & Corpse Medicine

Of Real Vampires, Gladiator Juice, a Not-So-Innocent Pope, Blood Marmalade, Skull Moss, and Mummy Remedies

The year was 1758. James and Walter White, ages twenty-three and twenty-one, were set to be executed by hanging at Kennington Common, in London. Hangings were a wonderful way to remind people not to commit crimes and, moreover, were an excellent source of entertainment. Like many executions at the time, the criminals were likely driven up to the gallows in a cart, their necks encircled with stout rope that would be bound to the high beam set up in the common. In short order, the cart would be pulled away and those who were once criminals would swing and jerk in the breeze until they were lifeless corpses.

While the bodies hung, the April 1758 issue of *The Gentleman's Magazine* reported, "a child, about nine months old was put into the hands of the executioner, who nine times, with one of the hands of each of the dead bodies, stroked the child over the face." The child suffered from *wens*, growths on the skin (likely boils). And the hope was that the dead men could cure them.

This might seem grotesque, but the use of human body parts for medicinal purposes had been popular since ancient Greece and Rome, spanning the Middle Ages and dying out (ha!) before the twentieth century. Corpses were sought after, and not just for touching, but for eating, drinking, and so much more. Call it cannibalism, call it anthropophagy, call it corpse medicine. Take your pick.

Throughout history, people have sought to consume what they crave— youth, vitality, strength. For many of the greatest standard-bearers in medicine, consuming pieces of dead humans fit into their philosophies of restoring health. The Galenic model of humors supported the idea that too much blood might be bad, but too little might be fixed with a long drink of the fluid. Hippocrates mentioned the use of something polluting—"corpse-food" or the "polluted blood of violence" (i.e., criminals' blood)—to fight impurity or disease. And later, Paracelsus thought that human-containing remedies healed via the "spirits" and essences within. A simple magical touch worked, too. In the seventeenth century, Robert Fludd noted that "A dead bodies hand touching warts, they will dye." Jan Baptiste van Helmont, a Flemish scientist and physician around the same time, believed the human corpse held "an obscure vitality," that the life force somehow lingered in the blood and body, particularly if the corpses had died a violent death. In other words, no energy had been wasted on a lingering illness or debility. This was why criminals who met untimely ends were such a hot commodity.

For the sake of this discussion, we'll focus on the use of the body and blood, unwillingly taken, for the most part. Of course, there were recipes for urine, essays on breastmilk for adults, fecal poultices, elixirs of sweat, and placenta pill discussions aplenty—but these somewhat "excretionary" items can be given without harm to the giver.

Blood, too, can be given without harm. After all, humans have generously donated it in the last century to save countless lives. But the use of blood in the past was not so clean or altruistic. It was a bloody mess.

BLOOD JAM AND OTHER VAMPIRE SNACKS

We tend to think of vampires as bloodsuckers endowed with gleaming canines and seductive charm, but in reality, humans who drank blood were an altogether less glamorous sort. In the first century, Pliny the Elder wrote that "the blood of gladiators is drunk by epileptics as though it were the draught of life," a perfect example of the sick desiring the prime health of

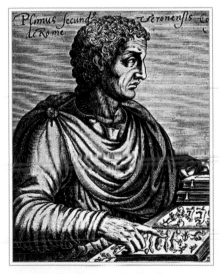

Pliny the Elder thinks you should suck on two gladiators and call him in the morning.

a fine, muscular specimen of humanity. Why blood? It's not clear, but when scholar after scholar insists that "It works because I heard it works," then people believe it. Ah, the power of the anecdote! Furthermore, epileptic seizures are often episodic. It would be easy to believe that any medicine was effective when someone went seizure-free for a few months after a dose.

Blood was the noblest of the humors, and also coined *elixir vitae*, or the elixir of life. Fifteenth-century Italian scholar Marsilio Ficino thought that young blood could restore vigor to the elderly. They should "suck, there-fore, like leeches, an ounce or two from a scarcely opened vein of the left arm. . . ." Oh, but what if you think drinking blood is repugnant? Then, Ficino advised, you should "let [the blood] first be cooked together with sugar, or let it be mixed with sugar and moderately distilled over hot water and then drunk."

Those who didn't have dead gladiators at their disposal had to be more resourceful. An Englishman named Edward Browne witnessed several exe-cutions in Vienna in the winter of 1668. After one beheading, he watched "a man run speedily with a pot in his hand, and filling it with blood, yet spouting out of [the corpse's] neck, he presently drank it off." Others dipped handkerchiefs into the blood, hoping to cure themselves of epilepsy, or as they called it, "the falling sickness."

And the stories go on.

But if there's any validity to the old adage that "the truth is stranger than fiction," then perhaps one story—unconfirmed—is wild enough to be real. In 1492, Pope Innocent VIII was on his deathbed. He wasn't exactly a saint. An unscrupulous politician, he depleted the papal treasury through his squabbles with Italian states, fathered sixteen illegitimate children, and dabbled in witch persecution and slavery. Not exactly a lovely guy to begin with. Rumor had it that, as a last resort, his physician bribed three young boys with a gold coin each. They were bled copiously and the ailing pope drank their blood. The boys died. The pope died. And the physician had a ter-rible reputation afterward (some say the rumor was spread as an anti-Semitic smear campaign against the physician). Could Pope Innocent VIII, a man with enormous power and dubious morals, have allowed the slaying of a few youths in a desperate attempt to stay alive? Perhaps.

Human blood wasn't just drunk. It was also dried, ground to a powder, and mixed into foods and ointments and sniffed up the nostrils. Italian doc-tor Leonardo Fioravanti thought blood products could "as good as raise the dead." He died in 1588, so it probably didn't work for him. Pliny described how the Egyptian kings attempted to cure their parasitic infections, which caused massive swelling called elephantiasis, by bathing in human blood. Blood was used for skin infections, fevers, and to make hair grow. Elsewhere in Europe, blood was sometimes cooked down into a sticky jam. Yes. Blood Jam. Wondering how to whip up a batch? A 1679 recipe from a Franciscan apothecary shows how:

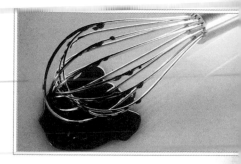

1. Let the blood dry into a sticky mass.
2. Cut it into thin slices and let the watery part drip away.
3. Stir it into a batter on the stove with a knife.
4. Pound it through a sieve of the finest silk, then seal in a glass jar.

They don't mention if it should be eaten on toast, or scones. But they do tell you where to get the blood: from a person with a "blotchy, red complexion." Actually, redheaded victims' blood was especially sought after. Weasley lovers of the world, look away. We beg you.

A BRIEF HISTORY OF EATING HUMANS FOR HEALTH

Pity those gingers. Another recipe for redheaded cadavers comes from a German physician in the early 1600s. "Choose the carcass of a red man, whole, clear without blemish, of the age of twenty-four years, that hath been hanged, broke upon a wheel, or thrust-through." The flesh should then be chopped to bits, sprinkled with herbs like myrrh and aloe, and mashed in wine. Afterward, it was dry-cured in a shady spot, where it would become comparable to smoked meat "without stink." If you're envisioning beef jerky, then you've got the right idea, though eating the jerky wasn't the end point. A red tincture would then be obtained from the dried flesh, and used as a restorative wound treatment or for a slew of other ailments.

This brings us to anthropophagy—the consumption of humans. When those gladiators fell, people drank a pint or so of blood, but they also ate the athletes' raw, fresh livers, again hoping to cure epilepsy. Liver was often considered an organ where courage resided, and replete with useful blood. Puritan Edward Taylor (d. 1729), Harvard graduate and rather famous for his poetry, was less known for his medical "Dispensatory." In it, he described how the dead human body contained a wealth of cures for the living. The marrow of bones was good for cramps. Gallbladder "relieveth in Deafness." Dried heart cured epilepsy. And the list goes on.

Then there was the possibility of candied humans. The legend of the "honeyed man," or mellified man, comes from the text of a sixteenth-century Chinese pharmacologist named Li Shizhen. He wrote of a rumor that there was an Arabian practice of mummifying a human with honey. Apparently the body had to come voluntarily from an elderly person. Without the self-sacrifice, the medicine would be useless. The volunteer would eat nothing but honey for days and days, until their excrement became honey, their sweat became honey, and they urinated honey (totally not possible, but hey, it's a legend). And then after dying (as one would, eventually), the body would be entombed in a coffin filled with honey. After exactly one hundred years, the embalmed body would then be consumed, piece by sweet piece. Who wouldn't want a piece of candied man? Actually, don't answer that.

Honey is a fantastic antibacterial and preservative, and has been used for medicinal purposes in cultures for centuries. So perhaps combining it with corpse medicine made some sort of morbid confectionary sense. Of course, there's no evidence that "mellified men" ever existed, but given the history of medical cannibalism, one wonders.

THE HEALING POWER OF "MAN'S GREASE"

Corpses were not just for a bloody drink or a curing touch. Executioners made a pretty penny off the skin and fat of dispatched criminals. Apothecaries were particularly fond of "oil of human fat," also called man's grease, poor sinner's fat, and hangman's salve. It was employed for wound healing, pain relief, cancers, love potions, gout, and rheumatism. An old German rhyme stated, "Melted human fat is good for lame limbs. If one rubs them with it, they become right again." Fat was also touted as a cure for hydrophobia (fear of drinking water), often synonymous with rabies. "Man's grease" could even be used in cosmetics, particularly if you had smallpox scars, and it was considered a great anti-inflammatory salve.

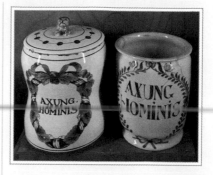

The executioners who dealt in death also recommended that human skin could help pregnant women—yep, they were their own brand of grim reaper/apothecary, and no one doubted the purity of their products. Some women believed that wearing tanned skin around their bellies helped childbirth pains. Human skin could also be worn around the neck to prevent goiters, or thyroid enlargement. One executioner's wife used human fat to treat a woman's broken hand in the 1700s. And in colonial America, physician Edward Taylor—he of the disturbingly resourceful approach to medical cannibalism—believed that skin cured "Hystericall Passions."

What can we say? It really makes your skin crawl. You need a thick skin to read this. Grease is the word? Okay, we'll stop now.

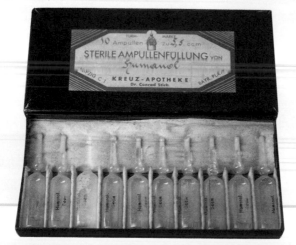

*Above: Seventeenth-
or eighteenth-century
apothecary vessels
for human fat.
Left: Ampules of human
fat.*

FOOD FOR YOUR NOGGIN (OR VICE VERSA)

Take the brains of a young man that has died a violent death,
together with the membranes, arteries, and veins, nerves . . . and
bruise these in a stone mortar until they become a kind of pap.
Then put as much of the spirit of wine as will cover it . . . [then]
digest it half a year in horse dung.

Recipe for "Essence of Man's Brains" from
The Art of Distillation (1651), John French

This recipe—for a bottle of brains and wine aged in a pile of warm, decomposing horse shit—is just one of many attempts to treat epilepsy using brains and skulls. Much of the logic behind medical cannibalism came from the homeopathic "like cures like" theory, so the brain and skull were paramount to curing ills thought to stem from the head itself. Many thought the skull was particularly important; as Flemish physician Jan Baptist van Helmont described it, after death "all the brain is consumed and dissolved in the skull" and "acquires such virtues."

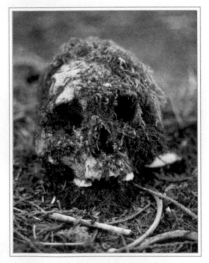

Seventeenth-century prescription for a bloody nose: Scrape some moss off a skull and stuff it up your nostrils.

From the ancient Greeks, who reportedly used pills of dead man's brains, to Christian IV of Denmark, who was said to treat himself with powdered skull, the battle against epilepsy, also known as "fits," was fought using the brain itself. Given that practitioners (correctly) assumed that epileptic symptoms were due to a brain ailment, the cure sort of made sense. Besides the powdered state, skulls were also shaved like ginger root, or sometimes used as a vessel to drink water. If you drank wine out of the bejeweled and silver-encrusted skulls of St. Theodul or St. Sebastian, you might cure your fits and fever.

From the seventeenth through nineteenth centuries, skulls were often found hanging for sale in chemists' shops in England and throughout Europe. And one's macabre medicine cabinet wouldn't be complete without some skull moss. A fluffy, greenish moss that grew on a skullcap exposed to the elements for long periods of time, the moss was rumored to stop a nosebleed when stuffed up your nostrils. So would a wadded up tissue, but anyway.

King Charles II of England (see Bloodletting, page 129), who dabbled in chemistry himself in the seventeenth century, purchased a particular recipe from a chemist named Jonathan Goddard. The elixir was known both as "spirit of skull" and for years as "Goddard's drops," but after Charles II purchased the recipe, it was most famously known as "the king's drops." Its recipe came down to cooking pieces of skull in a glass container. After much processing, the resulting distilled liquid could be used as a panacea, but most specifically for gout, heart failure, swelling, and epilepsy. One sad lady named Anne Dormer wrote in 1686 that when she felt unrested, restless, and meek, she took "the king's drops and [drank] chocolate." Thanks, but we'd rather have the chocolate.

In the 1700s, recommendations for spirit of human skull abounded for swoonings, apoplectic attacks, and nervous fits. The king's drops were used until the Victorian era, when they faded from pharmacoepias. After all, the product's reputation seemed to inconveniently lack one important point. On his deathbed, Charles II took his own king's drops in an effort to cure himself, and, well, he died.

OH, MUMMY

Speaking of the dead from long, long ago, one item found in European materia medica for hundreds of years was an ingredient called *mumia*. That's right. Mummies. Whether this ingredient actually came from real Egyptian mummies depends on the item, period of time, and, in some cases, etymology. Let's discuss.

An early Arabic medicine ingredient was mineral pitch called *mumiya*, from the Persian word *mūm*, or wax. It's a sticky, sometimes semisolid black form of petroleum that was used for poultices and antidotes. Around the eleventh century, people began to misidentify another supposed source of this mineral pitch, a dark substance found in the head and body cavities of ancient Egyptian embalmed bodies. Called *mummia* or *mumia*, it soon became synonymous with the entire embalmed corpse or any products that came from it.

What did minerals from a mummy skull taste like? A London pharmacopoeia in 1747 described it as "acrid and bitterish." Thank goodness. Because if it tasted like a Boston cream doughnut, heads would spin.

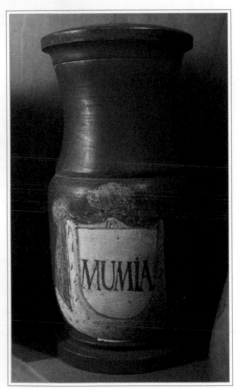

Mumia from mummies was in high demand at its peak in popularity in fifteenth- and sixteenth-century Europe, partly from being understood as "the sovereign remedy" according to Paracelsus. The physician and his followers believed that the body's spirit could be physically distilled into its highest form and that this "quintessence" could cure almost anything. Well, not really—there's no biological basis for it working. But Paracelsan medical cannibalism surged ahead anyway and became

Eighteenth-century apothecary jar.

an entirely acceptable practice, with *mumia* at its center. Physicians claimed it could cure ulcers, tumors, spitting up blood, bruising, gout, plague, poisoning, ringworm, and migraines. Did you drop your phone into the toilet? Maybe *mumia* could fix that, too.

Mummy-infused poultices were used to heal snakebites, syphilitic sores, headaches, jaundice, joint pain, and, yet again, epilepsy. In 1585, French royal surgeon Ambroise Paré exclaimed that when it came to healing bruises, mummy was "the first and last medicine of almost all our practitioners."

The demand led to a lively and sometimes illicit trade. Tombs in Cairo were raided and the corpses boiled to retrieve the oily substance floating at the top. Mummy heads were sold for gold. There was even a mummy import tax in England. Hundreds of pounds of mummy parts were sold to London apothecaries. Some thought that the ingredients used to embalm the mummies—ointments, aloes, myrrh, saffron—added to the mystique and richness of the source.

After much plundering, mummies became scarce. Counterfeits began to show up in the form of other bodies—beggars, lepers, and plague victims, their corpses scavenged and then stuffed with aloes, myrrh, and bitumen, then baked or dried in a furnace and dipped in pitch. Buyers didn't know any better but were advised to "choose what is of a shining black, not full of bones and dirt, and of a good smell." The need for mummies expanded to include those unfortunate travelers who perished in the African desert from deadly sandstorms. Called "Arabian mummies," these corpses were naturally embalmed by the dry environment.

Thankfully, the mummy trade dried up in the late eighteenth century. Once Paracelsan logic began to fail with modern physicians, *mumia* products faded. Medical knowledge progressed and the magical qualities of the human body were replaced by rational anatomical truths. Disgust—and the fact that *mumia* didn't work—certainly played a part, too.

DON'T EAT WHAT YOU ARE

The "hangman's stroke" ended in England in April 1845. They might not have known it at the time, but those lucky few women at the execution were the last to have their wens rubbed by a corpse (at least legally). The scene was described to be as "extraordinary as it was revolting to behold."

Ingestion of corpses, cooking brains, and sucking blood are all unthinkable today. And yet it's commonplace and quite acceptable to use other people's body parts for medicinal reasons. Organ donation and organ transplantation are miracles come true. Blood transfusions occur daily. And we are getting smaller and smaller in our focus when using other people's bodies—stem cells, bone marrow, and donation of eggs and sperm, for example. We borrow other people's wombs for surrogacy. And yet, plenty of people squirm at the idea of breastmilk banks. We are a society of contradictions.

Occasional horrifying articles pop up about "fetal pills" smuggled in from China, aiming to boost stamina and cure any manner of ills. Stories of stolen organs for black market transplantation still lurk about. Luckily in the United States, the laws are on the side of the deceased to honor their wishes about organ donation and not allow them to mysteriously end up in someone's medicine cabinet.

But it is no wonder that humans have looked to themselves—literally—to cure everything gone wrong. The desperate search to find health sometimes brings the best—and the worst—out of humanity.

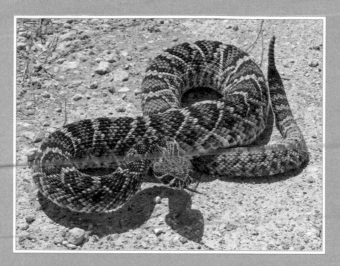

21

Animal-Derived Medicines

Of the Original Snake Oil Salesman, Ox Brains, and All Sorts of Testicles

In all the hustle and bustle of the 1893 Columbian Exposition in Chicago, a place where John Philip Sousa's band played nightly, the first electric kitchen was on display, and Pabst Blue Ribbon made its debut, Clark Stanley needed to make an impression.

Dressed to the nines in a showy, frontiersman fashion, Stanley stood on a stage in front of the massing crowd and reached into a sack at his feet. He pulled out a rattlesnake, showing the audience its writhing, venomous body, then deftly slit the snake open with his knife and plunged it into a vat of boiling water behind him. As the snake fat rose to the surface, Stanley skimmed it off, mixed it into previously prepared liniment jars, and sold it to the crowd as "Clark Stanley's Snake Oil Liniment."

The crowd in attendance for Stanley's debut at the fair were probably the only purchasers of his snake oil—and there would be thousands over the coming years—who actually had snake parts in their product. Stanley's liniment, as federal investigators would discover twenty-four years later, typically contained a lot less snake. As in none at all.

The official inquiry finally revealed the contents: mineral oil, beef fat, red pepper, and turpentine. Although that was good news for rattlesnakes, it was bad news for Stanley's many consumers, who had been duped by the world's first snake oil salesman.

In 1897, Stanley published an autobiography that was part self-mythology, part cowboy poetry, and part advertisement promoting his own snake oil. In *The Life and Adventures of the American Cowboy: Life in the Far West*, Stanley claimed to have learned of the great and mysterious healing powers of snake oil from the Hopi tribe.

Although it's a masterful origin story for Stanley, the self-dubbed "Rattlesnake King," the truth was more complicated.

During the wave of Chinese immigration to the American West in the 1800s, Americans were alternately repelled and intrigued by traditional Chinese medicinal practices. Snake oil was a popular, and legitimate, topical medicine used by Chinese laborers to relieve pain, reduce inflammation, and treat arthritis and bursitis. Chinese snake oil, made with the fat of Chinese water snakes—high in omega-3 fatty acids—was actually an effective anti-inflammatory.

But the problem with Chinese water snakes is they all live in China. So, once you run out of the snake oil you brought with you across the Pacific Ocean, what do you do next? You look for a local snake. And if you're anywhere west of the Rockies, that local snake is likely to have a rattle on its tail.

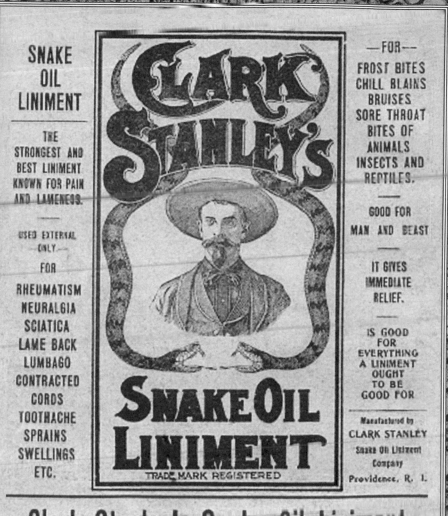

Rattlesnakes, unfortunately, contain much less beneficial fatty acids, about three times less than your average Chinese water snake. So snake oil made from rattlesnakes was not nearly as effective.

What was even less effective, however, was Stanley's Snake Oil Liniment because it contained no snake oil at all. It didn't matter. The "Rattlesnake King" was a master at self-promotion (when a reporter visited him in Massachusetts, he made sure to have his office filled with snakes, crawling all over the room and even up his arms), and he went happily about his business for two decades, making a tidy fortune. He even saw a good eleven years in operation after the Pure Food and Drug Act of 1906 began putting many of his quack colleagues out of business. The feds didn't catch up with Stanley until 1917, when they seized a shipment of his snake oil liniment, analyzed the contents, and issued their damning report.

Stanley was charged a whopping $20 fine for violating the Pure Food and Drug Act by "misbranding" his product.

He paid the fee, shrugged his shoulders, and slipped out of the pages of history a wealthy man.

INSANE IN THE MEMBRANE, INSANE IN THE OX BRAIN

Stanley was hardly the first quack to reach for the nearest animal, gut it, and advertise its contents as a panacea. Over the past few millennia, for both legitimate and illegitimate medical purposes, we've been crushing, testing, butchering, and torturing animals. This process of using animal products in medicine is called "zootherapy," but it's no trip to the zoo. Occasionally, animal research has led to significant, even crucial, discoveries. The fruit fly played a critical role in Thomas Hunt Morgan's early studies of genetics, Ivan Pavlov demonstrated the relationship between sense stimulation and body functions with his dogs, and Edward Jenner developed the first smallpox vaccine from cows (and promptly coined the term *vaccination* from the Latin *vacca* for "cow"). We've also employed animals to aid our own healing processes: Leeches, for example (see Leeches, page 211), were for many years considered an important weapon in the medicinal arsenal, snails have long been effective at healing burns, spiderwebs can be used to bind a wound, and, even today, maggots are used to clean out wounds.

But for every cow that helped humanity avoid smallpox, a few thousand died in the name of quackery. For example, take this prescription for insanity from the Renaissance era:

> Bake a loaf of bread, then remove the inner part and replace with an ox brain. Bind this ox-brain-filled bread to the patient's head. Insanity cured.

Yep, that ox just died so a mentally ill person could put its brain on his head.

The bit of sympathetic magic on display here (i.e., put the sedate brain of an ox near the unwell brain of a person) steered many animals toward untimely deaths, while simultaneously not working at all on the humans they were trying to cure.

Nevertheless, we have maintained a stubborn belief throughout the centuries in the power of sympathetic magic to overcome our medical trials. If the animal is strong, it will pass its strength on to us. If the animal is wise, it will pass its wisdom on to us.

And if the animal is virile, it will pass its virility on to us. And what's the most virile part of a virile animal?

Why, the testicles of course.

A TALE OF TWO TESTES

"Do you wish to continue as a sexual flat tire?" asked advertisements in the 1930s. If not, turn to "Doctor" John Romulus Brinkley, who offered a particularly jaw-dropping solution to the age-old problem of male impotence.

Brinkley—against all manner of reason and logic—convinced an embarrassingly large number of men that all they needed to restore their male virility was a new set of testicles. Goat testicles, to be exact.

Brinkley cut open the man's testicle sac, implanted slivers of goat testicles, then sewed the patient back up again. And so sexual flat tires were pumped back up and Brinkley became a multimillionaire.

The American quack was following on the heels of Serge Voronoff, a Russian-born physician practicing in France and Egypt in the early part of the twentieth century. Voronoff became convinced early in his medical career that the aging process was sped along by decreased hormonal activity. If instead you could increase hormone production, or rejuvenate aging glands, perhaps you could reverse the aging process.

At the relatively young age of thirty-three, Voronoff, in a valiant display of self-experimentation, injected himself with the ground-up testicles of castrated dogs and guinea pigs to see if it would halt his own aging process. It didn't.

Despite the complete lack of success, the experiment somehow convinced Voronoff the principle was sound. So, beginning in 1913, the physician turned to the ape family, transplanting the testicles from a baboon into the aging scrotum of a seventy-four-year-old man.

To be fair, Voronoff didn't actually overload the poor man's scrotum with full-size baboon testicles. Aware that such a surgery would invariably lead to the human body rejecting the foreign material, the physician came up with a more restrained strategy. He transplanted "slithers" of baboon testicles that measured two centimeters by half a centimeter. The thin slithers could thereby be absorbed by the human tissue, he reasoned, and the rejuvenation process could begin. The absorption part is true, the rejuvenation process . . . less so. The tissue died and the medical results were nonexistent. The placebo effect, however, was powerful.

BEAVER TESTICLES AND AMBERGRIS

Few items were more coveted for medieval medical dispensaries than beaver testicles and ambergris. Both male and female beavers excrete a yellow fluid called "castoreum" from their castor sacs, a type of scent gland. For the beavers, castoreum is useful for marking their territory. For humans, well, we've been convinced that castoreum is useful for pretty much every medical condition at some point in history. We were also convinced castoreum was found inside the beaver's testicles. (Hot tip: It's not.)

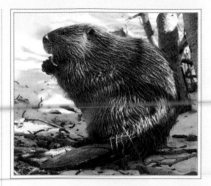

A beaver getting ready to throw his nuts at you.

We were so into beaver-testicle harvesting that a popular medieval legend was that beavers, weary from being hunted, would just chew off their testicles at the sight of humans and throw the newly freed body parts directly at their oppressors. While the folktale does give beavers an enviable degree of badassery, it's also totally bogus.

Ambergris, an excreted substance from the intestines of the sperm whale, has, like castoreum, been exploited by both perfume makers and physicians. The rare substance, roughly akin in value per weight to gold, was thought to be an effective medieval panacea, curing headaches, colds, heart disease, and epilepsy, for starters. You could even carry a ball of ambergris as a plague preventer (if you could afford to buy one).

Voronoff labeled the operation a success, and some seven hundred physicians present at London's International Congress of Surgeons in 1923 "oohed" and "ahhed" when Voronoff presented his new surgical techniques, adding a surprising air of temporary legitimacy to Voronoff's totally wacky claims. The surgeon professed that successful transplantation led to an increase in sex drive (that perennial male aging problem that has been exploited by quacks for centuries), as well as increased energy, better eyesight, and longer life.

Meanwhile, the Roaring Twenties were afoot and the global mood among the wealthy was one of unrestrained optimism and a gleeful willingness to experiment with new ideas. It was exactly the right time and place for monkey gland surgery to find a cultural foothold. Or rather, if there was ever the right time and place for monkey testicle transplantation, it was the 1920s. Monkey gland transplants became all the rage among the well-to-do and Voronoff became a fabulously wealthy celebrity surgeon, occupying the entire first floor of an expensive Paris hotel, attended to by a legion of valets and secretaries.

One surgeon noted that "fashionable dinner parties and cracker barrel confabs, as well as sedate gatherings of the medical elite, were alive with the whisper—'monkey glands.'" Voronoff performed his $5,000 surgery on somewhere between five hundred and one thousand men over the next decade, most commonly at a special clinic he'd established in Algiers. (The monkey testicles, by the way, were harvested from the animals kept at Voronoff's special "monkey farm" on the Italian Rivera.) Several notable people undertook the surgery, including Harold Fowler McCormick, chairman of the International Harvester Company, who hoped the procedure would help him keep up with his new, much younger wife, the Polish opera singer Ganna Walska. Another famous surgical participant was

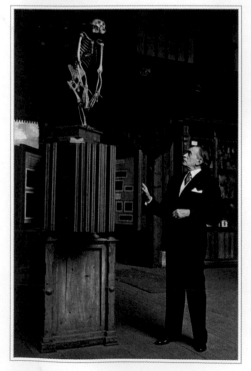

Voronoff exalting a chimpanzee.

Frank Klaus, a middleweight boxing champion who was fighting a losing battle against the onset of middle age.

Despite its popularity, as the 1920s rolled onward it became increasingly obvious that monkey gland surgery as male "enhancement" was a total bust. Voronoff drifted off into wealthy obscurity and when he died in 1951, few newspapers carried his obituary.

We suffer terribly from short-term memory, however, and it was only a scant few years after the downfall of the monkey gland that a new quack was advertising the rejuvenating abilities of the testicle from another creature entirely: the goat.

And now we return to John Romulus Brinkley. Instead of enrolling in a medical school sanctioned by the American Medical Association, Brinkley had opted for a cheaper, quackier route—the Eclectic Medical University in Kansas City. Brinkley was looking for fame and money, and the answer arrived with a resounding bleat.

Randy goat nuts, when transplanted into men's scrotums, would surely restore male virility and youthfulness. They didn't, of course—the transplanted tissue was rejected by the body, but the results of the placebo effect were once again surprisingly potent. As for the patients who were permanently injured by a surgeon who didn't actually hold a medical license? Well, that part of the story was conveniently swept under the rug.

MONKEY GLANDS

The monkey gland surgeries also made a deep cultural imprint in the 1920s, leading to a satirical novel (Mikhail Bulgakov's *Heart of a Dog*), a famous cocktail, and a Marx Brothers song in the film *The Cocoanuts*:

> Let me take you by the hand
> Over to the jungle band
> If you're too old for dancing
> Get yourself a monkey gland.

The Monkey Gland Cocktail Recipe

Created by famous mixologist Harry MacElhone, a standard Monkey Gland contains the following:

1½ ounces gin • 1½ ounces orange juice
1 teaspoon grenadine • 1 teaspoon absinthe

Shake, strain, and serve.

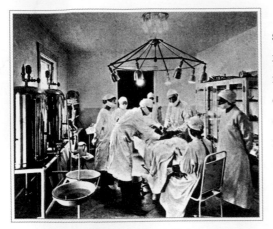

"Nurse, hand me the goat testicles." Brinkley's surgery in action.

Brinkley took his goat show on the road, touring nationally and internationally in the 1930s. His claims were called "rot" by a former president of the AMA. When asked in court how he knew his surgeries worked, Brinkley replied, "I can't explain it… I don't know." (Never words you want to hear from someone you're paying to slice into your scrotum.)

Despite his nonstop ambition (he came close to winning a bid for governor of Kansas, and opened up a wildly successful radio station on the Mexico border), Brinkley died bankrupt in 1942 after a flurry of lawsuits.

The Relative Civility of the Modern Era

As Western medicine developed in the early modern era, we came to rely less and less on slaughtering animals for elaborate cures, instead contenting ourselves with simply locking animals in cages and using them for medical experimentation. It was much more "civilized" that way.

But we haven't completely cut out animals from our drugs. Indeed, the dedicated vegan frequently finds himself in a quandary. Lest we feel too superior to our ancestors, here are some twenty-first-century cures rendered medieval style:

Diabetes Extract the pancreatic secretions of a hog, freshly killed, and inject into a vein in your arm. (insulin)

Dry eyes Extract the oil from the skin glands of a sheep and apply to eyes. (lanolin)

General illness Powder a variety of medical ingredients. Boil the bones, ligaments, and tendons of a cow or pig, and create a capsule from resulting mixture. Fill the capsule with medical ingredients, encourage patient to swallow. (gelatin)

Post-menopausal hot flashes Drink the urine of an impregnated mare. (Premarin)

Prevent blood clotting Extract mucus from the intestinal membranes of slaughtered pigs or from the lungs of slaughtered cows. Inject. (heparin)

So, really, we aren't all that different from our ancestors, and some of our modern-day cures derived from animals may well find themselves a target for quackery books in the future. Our medieval forebearers were on to something with the spiderwebs and the snail slime. But binding ox brains to the heads of the mentally ill? Not so much. In the future we may feel the same about impregnating mares to harvest their urine.

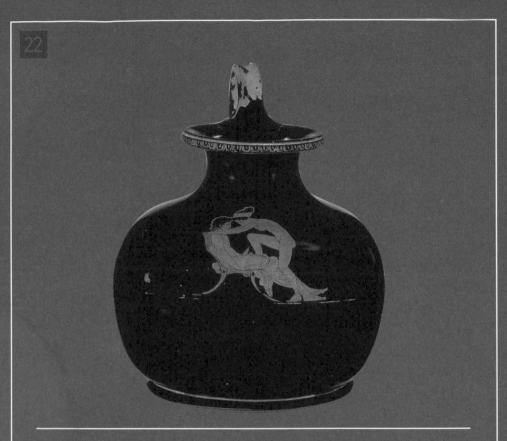

22

Sex

Of Grecian Orgies, Pelvic Massage Prescriptions, Rectal Dilators, the Orgone Box, and Spanking Your Way to Fertility

Remember the song "Sexual Healing" by Marvin Gaye? Well, Mr. Gaye was articulating in his oh-so-irresistible fashion an ancient sentiment that sex could be therapeutic. Not just procreating or expressing love or passing the time on a boring Sunday afternoon, but bona fide healing of the body. Although it took musical genius to spread this groovy message to the masses, the idea actually goes back several millennia.

For everything from hysteria to hemorrhoids, sexual activity has been prescribed for thousands of years as a cure. In roughly equal doses, however, abstinence has also been prescribed as a cure . . . often for the same diseases. We've rarely known what we were talking about. It's always been difficult for us to extract our politics and biases from our sexual diagnoses. But we're getting better. Slowly.

The zenith of medical intrusion into the bedroom was in the nineteenth century, when the Victorians, in a mind-boggling display of psychological hypocrisy, simultaneously encouraged female masturbation (via physicians) while condemning male masturbation. Our always complex medical relationship to our most intimate act, however, stretches even further back to the mountain slopes of ancient Greece.

An Orgy with The 300

Melampus was a rock star healer who shows up from time to time in ancient Greek mythology. One day, Melampus was called in by the ruler of Argos. The city was in the midst of a little problem: All of its virgins, after refusing to honor the phallus in a religious ritual, had gone mad and fled to the mountains. Melampus said, "No worries," and then tracked down the roving packs of virgins on the slopes, subduing the lot with hellebore and encouraging them to have sex with the strong young men of Greece. (Remember the bro-fest of a movie that was The 300? Yeah, Melampus was basically saying you'll feel a lot better if you have sex with guys who look like that.)

According to the story, Melampus's sage advice was heeded and actually worked. The women found their madness dissipated after getting it on with some hunky Greek warriors. They returned from the mountains and resumed their daily lives in Argos.

So what does this story really tell us? It's one of the first recorded instances of Western civilization encountering that age-old (male-created) issue of "female hysteria." Melampus's healing of the virgins was really an origin story for female madness stemming from a lack of sex. It was no accident, by the way, that Melampus went on to introduce the worship of Dionysus, god of fertility, to the rest of Greece. Feeling anxious, nervous, depressed, or in any way unfulfilled? Stop by a drunken orgy on Saturday night and you'll feel a lot better.

Hippocrates wrote quite extensively on hysteria, a term later coined in the nineteenth century. Basically placing all female health problems on the shoulders of a "wandering uterus," he declared that women could cure a whole host of illnesses through sex. The uterus, satisfied by sexual activity, would stop wandering around and making women sick. Bonus points if you got pregnant. But you had to be married. Virgins, widows, and single women were on their own. Hey, you can't heal everyone.

Hippocrates also thought that having sex would widen a woman's birth canal, leading to a cleaner and healthier body. He was kind of on the right track there. Recent research suggests that women who have wider birth canals, either by design or as a by-product of childbirth, often have less painful menstrual cramps.

In general, Hippocrates advocated that women get married and enjoy an active sex life to stay healthy. On the other hand, many doctors—namely Greece's Soranus and Rome's Galen—advocated abstinence for women's health. Of course, these were male doctors.

It would be another thousand years before women would be allowed to come to their own conclusions about their sexual health (much less actually practice medicine), but finally in eleventh-century Italy, we find Trota of Salerno, the first female doctor in medieval Europe. Trota was also the first writer to point out that sexual diseases were perhaps a bit intimate for female patients to discuss with their overwhelmingly male physicians. She viewed abstinence as a cause of illness and advised an active sex life within the bounds of marriage. She also recommended musk oil and mint to placate sexual desire, if need be. Musk oil and mint not your thing? Not to worry. Maybe the Victorians can offer something that's more your style.

SPANK YOUR WAY TO FERTILITY

According to Virgil, during the Roman feast of Lupercalia, basically a public orgy, naked men roamed the streets spanking any woman they came across. The Romans also believed that spanking a new bride—to the accompaniment of cymbals, no less—was a surefire way to guarantee her fertility. This belief even made its way into a Shakespeare play. In *Julius Caesar*, which starts off in the midst of a Lupercalia festival, Caesar himself instructs Mark Antony to "touch" (read: spank) his wife Calpurnia so that she will conceive:

> Forget not, in your speed, Antonius,
> To touch Calpurnia; for our elders say,
> The barren, touched in this holy chase,
> Shake off their sterile curse.

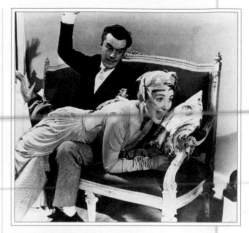

Man spanking woman in the hopes of producing an heir.

THE VICTORIANS TO THE RESCUE!

The notion of female hysteria likely reached its cultural zenith in the Victorian era, when women were repeatedly diagnosed with the condition for a wide array of generic symptoms, including fatigue, anxiety, and mild depression. The epidemic reached such epic levels during the second half of the nineteenth century that Dr. Russell Trall, a hydrotherapist, made the bold declaration that 75 percent of women in the United States suffered from hysteria. The cure? A "pelvic massage" of enough vigor to eventually induce a "hysterical paroxysm." The Victorians were masters at the pseudonym. Indeed, according to some historians, women were prescribed genital massages—conducted by their male doctors (!)—to induce orgasm.

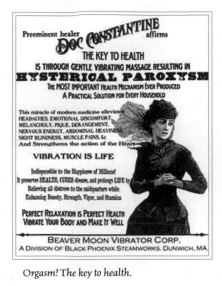

Orgasm! The key to health.

"Why, I say, Doctor, this all seems a bit . . . forward."

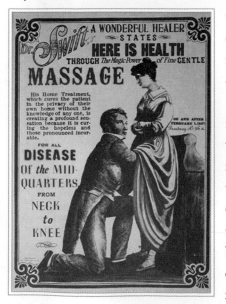

Now, you'd think that this might be part of some sort of large-scale mass delusion with a Freudian wet dream of sexual undertones. But here's the kicker: Physicians didn't think there was anything sexual about their "pelvic massages." In fact, they were kind of annoyed at having to do them at all. Doctors complained that the correct technique was very difficult to learn and was time consuming to boot. Some exhausted physicians reported a pelvic massage took about an hour to successfully perform and led to cases of "wrist-ache."

Lest we pity our poor Victorian doctors, laboriously massaging the genitals of their female patients, an important invention was about to come to their rescue: the electromechanical vibrator.

This device was no joke. Weighing in at forty pounds, it was powered by a wet cell battery and came with an assortment of little add-ons called "vibratodes." Invented by Dr. Joseph Mortimer Granville in the late nineteenth century, the vibrators were a hit with doctors because they reduced the time needed to obtain an orgasm from an hour to about five minutes.

Little did the physicians know, however, that they were cutting themselves out of the picture. As soon as vibrators became even remotely portable, a burgeoning kitchen industry in the manufacture and sale of household vibrators sprang onto a fertile market. Soon, the

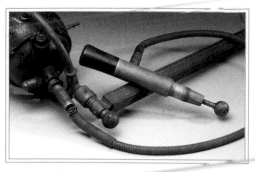

Steampunk vibrator.

modern woman of the early twentieth century could order a personal vibrator for a few dollars from the Sears catalog. It certainly beat paying your doctor to get you off, and it wasn't long before physicians stopped offering pelvic massages.

The vibrator was enormously popular, becoming the fifth electrical appliance introduced to the modern home. Let that sink in for a minute. Electricity comes along and pretty soon to keep up with the Joneses you needed a tea kettle, a sewing machine, a fan, a toaster, and . . . a vibrator.

The advertisements, which ran in all the leading women's magazines, as well as the general supply catalogs such as Sears, contained the wonderful hyperbole of the era: "The secret of the ages has been discovered in Vibration. Great scientists tell us that we owe not only our health but even our life strength to this wonderful force. Vibration promotes life and vigour, strength and beauty . . . Vibrate Your Body and Make It Well. YOU Have No Right to Be Sick."

Granville's vibrator (left) with battery. Hook her up to this contraption and see what happens next.

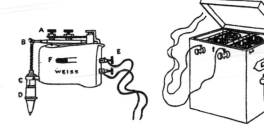

The concept of female hysteria as a diagnosable illness faded away as the twentieth century marched forward. Always something of a catchall diagnosis, as psychoanalytical techniques improved, hysteria diagnoses declined. In its place rose diagnoses of depression and anxiety, as well as cases of epilepsy, schizophrenia, personality disorder, and conversion disorder.

The wink-wink ruse of vibrators as strictly medical devices was ruined by early porn films in the 1920s introducing viewers to . . . nonmedical uses of them. The idea that vibrators were just oh-so-simple medical devices had run its course. The jig was up. Vibrators had moved firmly over to the sex toys side of the equation.

OTHER SEX TOYS IN THE MEDICINE CABINET

Of course, vibrators weren't the only sex toys on the market. In the 1890s, advertisements began cropping up in medical journals for Dr. Young's Ideal Rectal Dilators. Made of rubber and sold in sets of four that increased in size from one-half inch in diameter to four inches, the dilators were, well, Victorian butt plugs sold under the guise of health aids. The advertisements claimed that rectal dilators were particularly useful for cases of chronic constipation and piles (hemorrhoids), proclaiming, "If you will prescribe a set of these dilators in some of your obstinate cases of Chronic Constipation, you will find them necessary in every case of this kind." Priced at $2.50 "to the profession."

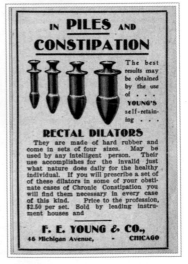

Dr. Young's Ideal Rectal Dilators were sold from the late nineteenth century until the 1940s, when the US Attorney for the

Rectal dilators come in a set of varying sizes so you may slowly broaden your, er . . . health benefits.

Southern District of New York seized a shipment of the devices for being mis-
leadingly labeled. No longer content with simply advertising the rectal dilators as constipation cures, the manufacturing company went on, in the usual
way of quacks, to add a seemingly endless series of medical claims to their
packaging. The company even promised to cure, of all things, foul breath and
bad tastes in the mouth. The instructions also boldly declared "Do not neglect
to use your Dilators . . . you need have no fear of using them too much."

The FDA disagreed, arguing that the claims that the dilators would permanently cure constipation and piles were not accurate. In fact, a dilator is
about the last thing you want to be messing with during a hemorrhoid attack.
The FDA also declared they were dangerous to health if used too frequently
or for too long. The shipment was destroyed, and Dr. Young's Ideal Rectal
Dilators ceased production. Don't worry, though, you can still find reproduc-
tions on the Internet.

THE ORGONE BOX

Not long after the downfall of rectal dilators, a psychologist with an entranc-
ing philosophy about sexual energy emerged to influence Western culture. Dr.
Wilhelm Reich, a member of the second wave of post-Freud psychoanalysts,
developed a complex theory about a universal life force he called "orgone," the
same universal life force acupuncturists might refer to as "qi," or simply "The
Force" to Star Wars enthusiasts. Reich argued that orgone was present in all living matter and that many diseases were the result of orgone flow being either
restricted or not available in sufficient quantities.

The best way to build and share orgone energy? Sex. As such, Reich
argued strongly for sexual liberation, tying it to complex philosophies about
the working-class revolution as well. He viewed the libido as an essential life-
affirming force that was constantly being repressed by the state.

Reich wasn't exactly a hit with conservatives.

He was a hit, however, with the budding countercultural movement in post–World War II America. The Beat Generation embraced his ideas and, particularly, his box. His orgone box. Reich's Orgone Institute built and sold (for donation only) "orgone boxes," also known as "orgone energy accumulators." They were basically large empty boxes that you would stand or sit in for hours at a time. They were built with alternating layers of organic and nonorganic materials inside the walls, which, we are told, increased the accumulation of orgone energy in the box. Feeling a bit depressed? Low on energy? You could simply sit inside your orgone box for a few hours, build up your orgone reserves, and feel a lot better again. They were also apparently a great way to accumulate sexual energy (i.e., increase orgone levels) by building up your libido through sitting for a long time and having your orgones reflected

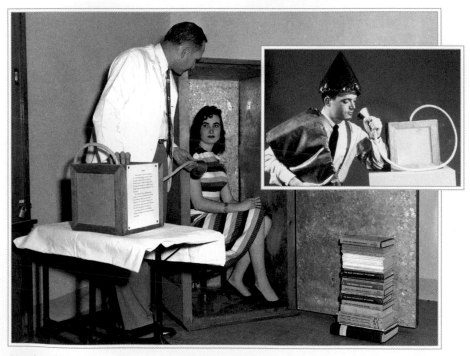

Now just sit in this box until you feel aroused.

JOHN HARVEY KELLOGG: PRO-CEREAL, ANTI-MASTURBATION

John Harvey Kellogg was a physician who founded a sanitarium in Battle Creek, Michigan, touting his way of healthy living. Name sound familiar? It's because he, along with his brother Will, invented Kellogg's Corn Flakes (originally called Granula). Kellogg's ideas for healthy eating and weight maintenance made some sense—plenty of exercise, no excessive calories, vegetarianism, and abstinence from alcohol and tobacco. Another thing Kellogg vehemently thought you should abstain from? Masturbation. He hated it and thought it was the unhealthiest thing you could possibly do for your body, mind, and soul. In his 1877 book, *Plain Facts for Old and Young*, Kellogg discusses in detail the evils of what he called "self-abuse" and "unchastity."

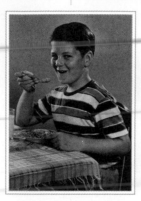

Diet was, predictably from the creator of Corn Flakes, one major way to cure masturbatory habits. He wrote, "A man that lives on pork, fine-flour bread, rich pies and cakes, and condiments, drinks tea and coffee, and uses tobacco, might as well try to fly as to be chaste in thought." Also, never overeat. "Gluttony is fatal to chastity," he wrote, also regarding all spices and pickles as evil. Apparently, a world without pickles is as unsexually stimulating as you can get.

Kellogg's predecessor, Sylvester Graham, claimed that white bread was devoid of nutrients and recommended a flour product without additives. The bread was soon made into crackers in 1829, eaten in great quantities by "Grahamites" who practiced the Graham Diet—vegetarian, with lots of whole wheat and high-fiber foods. Oh, and no alcohol. The crackers were part of a plan to fight urges to masturbate, as well. Those original Graham crackers were a bit different from the sugar-laden ones we eat at campfires, together with toasted marshmallows and chocolate. If Graham and Kellogg could eat our s'mores, based on that original chaste cracker, they'd have probably had a death-inducing orgasm.

back at you. Well, hey, after sitting in a box for four hours, sex undoubtedly felt pretty awesome.

Considering that we are literally talking about an empty box to sit in, the orgone boxes were surprisingly popular for a brief period of time. Albert Einstein was even lured into trying one out, but he quickly lost patience with the box—and with Reich's theories in general—after a short stint inside. William S. Burroughs, the author of *Naked Lunch*, however, was a dyed-in-the-wool convert. He built his own orgone box (technically against the rules, but Burroughs wasn't exactly a rule follower) and would spend hours inside as a way to reduce symptoms of "junk sickness" (i.e., heroin withdrawal). For that purpose, orgone boxes may indeed have worked quite well.

Burroughs even introduced Nirvana singer Kurt Cobain to an orgone box, and a photo floats around the Internet to this day of Cobain waving and smiling from the inside. The singer commented in 1993 that he had to have Burroughs kill all the spiders in the box, though, before he got in.

Eventually, Reich's health claims for his orgone boxes drew the attention—and wrath—of the FDA, who obtained a federal injunction barring distribution of orgone materials. Reich was also tossed in jail for continuing to distribute his research and products across state lines, and much of his orgone research was destroyed. If you want to sit in an orgone box today, you might need to make one yourself. (Don't worry, there are directions on the Internet.) Vintage orgone boxes from the Wilhelm Reich days are scarce, although you can still find one at the Reich Museum in Rangeley, Maine, if a trip to New England is in your future.

SEX IS GOOD FOR YOU

Even if you can't find an orgone box, physicians have shown that you can enjoy significant medical benefits from a healthy sex life. And you don't have to sit in a box for a few hours to build up your orgone levels first. Regular sex may improve your immune system, lower your blood pressure, improve your sleep, and lower your stress levels.

So grab your partner, blast some Marvin Gaye, and get it on.

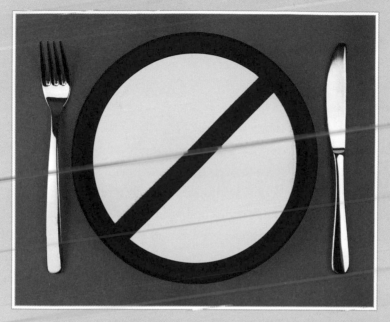

23

Fasting

Of Fasting Saints, Starvation Heights, the "Brooklyn Enigma," the Delicious Taste of Air, and the Deadly Past of a Popular Cleanse

The year 1908 was an important one in the life of "fasting specialist" Linda Hazzard. It was the year she authored her first book, *Fasting for the Cure of Disease*, which argued that fasting was a panacea for virtually every illness. It was also the first year a patient died under her supervision.

Hazzard claimed that toxins were at the root of all disease and needed to be expunged via fasting. Her sanatorium in Olalla, Washington, was quickly dubbed "Starvation Heights" by locals as rumors trickled down of enemas that lasted for hours, pummeling

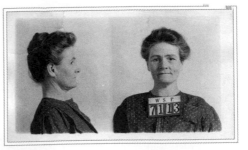

Linda Hazzard heading where she belonged.

massages, and diets that included nothing but miniscule amounts of tomato, asparagus, and orange juice for days on end. Although it may sound like the latest Goop-inspired celebrity fasting trend, it was actually a vicious, terrible dieting strategy, and a lot of people died from it. So don't get any ideas.

The first patient to die under her care was Norwegian immigrant Daisey Haglund, who passed away from starvation-related complications at the age of thirty-eight. (Historical trivia side note: Daisey's son, Ivar Haglund, who also had occasionally been subjected to Hazzard's treatments, went on to found Ivar's Seafood restaurants, a Seattle chain still in operation today. So order a huge meal next time you're at Ivar's in celebration of not starving yourself to death.)

Unfortunately, it would take four more years and the death of a wealthy British woman named Claire Williamson before the law finally caught up with Hazzard. Williamson's weight at the time of her death?

Fifty pounds.

As a grown woman.

Claire's sister, Dora, was still in Hazzard's care at the time of her death. She had also dropped to close to fifty pounds, a weight so low that sitting was painful for her. After her sister's death, Dora managed to smuggle out a telegram plea for help to her family. The younger Williamson was rescued from the sanatorium and Hazzard was brought up on charges of manslaughter.

At the subsequent trial, it became clear that Hazzard had forged Claire Williamson's will, while also helping herself to approximately $6,000 in jewelry from both sisters. It wasn't an isolated incident. At least fourteen other patients died under Hazzard's care, but not before she had either convinced them, in their weakened mental and physical states, to sign over their earthly possessions to her, or simply forged their wills herself.

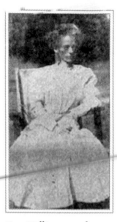

Hazzard was convicted, sentenced to two to twenty years in prison, and released on parole a paltry two years later. To add insult to injury, she managed to obtain a pardon from the governor of Washington. Although she was banned from practicing medicine again, she did open a "school of health" in Olalla, where she con-

Dora Williamson, whose weight had dropped close to fifty pounds.

tinued to espouse the fasting gospel until 1938 when she died of starvation while attempting a fasting cure herself. At least she practiced what she preached.

THE MIRACLE OF MALNOURISHMENT: FASTING ACROSS THE AGES

Hazzard had taken to a dangerous extreme a medical practice that, with some legitimacy, stretches back centuries.

In ancient Greece, Pythagoras argued that periodic fasting was good for the body. In the Renaissance era, Paracelsus referred to fasting as "the physician within." And the well-worn maxim of "feed a cold, starve a fever" has been traced to a 1574 dictionary by English lexicographer John Withals, who wrote, "Fasting is a great remedy of fever."

In moderation, Paracelsus was right: Fasting can be good for the body. Religious leaders throughout history also recognized that it can be good for the soul. Fasting as a spiritual practice sprang up independently across the globe as a means of preparation for religious rituals, or to invite ecstatic

THE CURIOUS CASE OF THE BROOKLYN ENIGMA

Mollie Fancher, aka "the Brooklyn Enigma," was diagnosed with dyspepsia in 1864 when she was sixteen years old and just a few months shy of graduation from the Brooklyn Heights Seminary. Fancher's dyspepsia symptoms, in addition to frequent fainting spells and a weakness of the chest, forced her to drop out of school.

Things only got worse from there. Later that year, Mollie was thrown from a horse, was knocked unconscious, and broke several ribs. A little more than a year later, her dress caught on the hook of a carriage, dragging her for a whole city block and once again knocking her unconscious and breaking several ribs.

Mollie never really recovered. She was put to bed to heal; her engagement fell apart; and she began manifesting a bizarre series of symptoms, eventually losing the majority of her senses, including sight, touch, taste, and smell. Either because of her illness or in an attempt to recover, Mollie also stopped eating. She reportedly went

a full sixteen years without consuming any food. Observers claimed that her stomach "collapsed, so that by placing the hand in the cavity her spinal column could be felt."

While lying in a supine position with her arm drawn over her head, her legs twisted beneath her, and her eyes closed, Mollie also claimed to be able to read minds, read writing from a great distance, and offer prophecies. In a country bewitched by the spiritualist movement, she was an overnight sensation. Between 1866 and 1875, stories repeatedly surfaced in the press about the wondrous spiritual abilities of the Brooklyn Enigma, and the case of Mollie Fancher was much debated in medical and societal circles.

Sometime in the late 1880s or early 1890s, Mollie apparently began eating food again, and, in turn, her strange symptoms began to disappear. (Reversing starvation is really a wonderful cure.)

Mollie lived on, without further incident, until 1916.

visions and dreams. Looking for a divine revelation? Fasting was seen across cultures as a pretty good way to get you there.

One of the first recorded people to combine fasting for spiritual enlightenment with fasting for medical treatment was Saint Lidwina. In Lidwina's time in the late fourteenth century, ice skating was still the primary method of travel along the Netherlands' frozen canals during winter. When she was fifteen years old, Lidwina took a bad spill while out on her skates. A really bad spill. So bad, in fact, that she never completely recovered, progressively becoming more and more disabled. (Today, Lidwina is generally thought to have been one of the earliest cases of multiple sclerosis.)

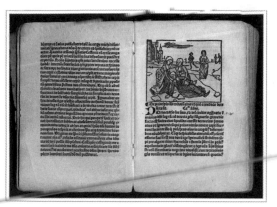

St. Lidwina's ice-skating accident.

In what began as an attempt to heal and quickly became laced with religious overtones, Lidwina began a hardcore fast, working her way down from apples, to dates, to watered wine, to river water contaminated with salt from the sea, to eventually breath alone. Her reputation grew as a healer and holy woman, and Dutch officials stationed guards around her to verify her claims of not eating anything at all. They agreed that she wasn't eating (and maybe even raped her while they were at it, according to some accounts). As Lidwina's disease progressed, she apparently dropped various body parts, which were quickly scooped up and used as religious idols.

Including her intestines.

Fasting continued to captivate people for centuries after St. Lidwina, spreading into the secular world with the rise of "fasting girls" in the Victorian era. Cases like Brooklyn's Mollie Fancher (see box "The Curious Case of the Brooklyn Enigma," opposite) and Wales's Sarah Jacobs quickly became international news. Originally fasting for healing purposes, both were transformed into overnight celebrities. (Ever heard the phrase "starving for attention"?) While Mollie resumed eating and eventually recovered, Sarah was not so lucky. Considered miraculous by the Welsh peasantry,

Sarah's case drew the attention of the press and inspired a round-the-clock guard by several local nurses to confirm that she actually was not eating. She must have been eating secretly because, under the strain of the 24-hour surveillance, Sarah lapsed into unconsciousness after four days, starving to death shortly after. Her parents were quickly convicted of manslaughter and shipped off to prison.

You'd think after such horror stories, humanity would have learned its lesson. But the quackery of fasting was just getting started.

A Plate of Air and Sunshine

Fasting got a boost in the late nineteenth century when several doctors on both sides of the Atlantic began advocating a set of health practices broadly referred to as "Natural Hygiene." With slight variances from practitioner to practitioner, the recommended healthy behaviors included eating a balanced diet, getting plenty of fresh air and exercise, taking in the sun, and drinking lots of water. So far, so good, right? But the Natural Hygiene movement also included recommendations for avoiding physician-prescribed drugs when sick and healing yourself through fasting.

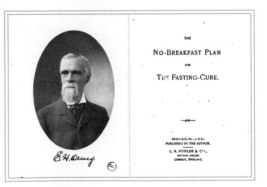

An entire book about not eating breakfast.

Dr. Edward Dewey, an American who practiced in the second half of the nineteenth century, was a leader in the therapeutic fasting movement. He outlined his vision for health in a book entitled *The No-Breakfast Plan*, which spread its way around the globe. *The No-Breakfast Plan* boiled health down to two basic principles: Don't eat breakfast (in case that wasn't obvious from the title) and don't eat when you're sick. Unless you're hungry.

Somehow Dewey stretched out those two simple points into many pages, mostly by filling them up with wordy testimonials from the hundreds of patients he claimed to have cured. Dewey also trained a variety of other young physicians in his methods. Including a young girl from Minnesota named Linda Hazzard.

When Hazzard wrote about Dewey's 1904 death, she criticized her old mentor for realizing the health benefits of the cinema too late in life. She also berated him for dying from paralysis because of an "error in personal dietary." Although Dewey strictly observed his touted No-Breakfast Plan, he ignored "food values, food adaptability, [and] food combination" in his two permitted daily meals. As a result, to Hazzard's great horror, "meats and fish, eggs and milk, breads and pastries, with comparatively few vegetables in combination, and these mostly of the starchier kinds, formed his food supply. What wonder that hardened veins, high blood pressure, and ultimate paralysis developed!" And so Hazzard provided the groundwork for her medical philosophy at Starvation Heights.

The Natural Hygiene movement was later co-opted into the "Nature Cure" in the twentieth century by Dr. Herbert Shelton, of "Dr. Shelton's Health School" fame, who purported to have cured more than forty thousand patients with water fasting.

Shelton wrote of his formative educational experiences: "I postgraduated from the University of Hard Knocks and left before I got my diploma. I went through the usual brainwashing process of the school system in Greenville, Texas and revolted against the whole political, religious, medical, and social system at the age of sixteen."

Shelton went on to obtain a "doctor of physiological therapeutics" (never heard of that degree?) from a bogus college established by Bernarr Macfadden. His first book, *The Fundamentals of Nature Cure*, arrived in 1920

THE DETOX BOX

Detoxing, a modified form of fasting aimed at removing toxins from the body, is the diet trend du jour. In a typical detox, you abstain from consuming food for a period of days, instead relying upon juices and/or water and/or specific supplements to sustain yourself. The Liver Cleanse, the 10-Day Green Smoothie Cleanse, the Colon Cleanse, the Blueprint Cleanse, and Slendera Garcinia Cambogia are all variations on this theme.

The most notorious cleanse, however, is the Master Cleanse, developed by Stanley Burroughs, which relies upon drinking a concoction of lemon water, maple syrup, and cayenne pepper, in conjunction with a detox tea, for ten days. Short-term side effects of the Master Cleanse include nausea, dehydration, dizziness, and fatigue. Long-term side effects of the Master Cleanse include . . . death. In fact, that's exactly what happened to one of Burroughs's patients in the 1980s. A cancer patient named Lee Swatsenbarg sought out medical advice from Burroughs, who recommended a thirty-day cleanse, combined with exposure to specific colors of light and intense massages.

Swatsenbarg took Burroughs up on his advice, embarking on a month-long detox wherein his health continually worsened and he began vomiting and suffering from severe convulsions. He died before he could complete the treatment, after suffering a massive hemorrhage in his abdomen thanks to the abdominal massages that Burroughs threw in (for an additional fee) on top of the detox plan. Burroughs was convicted on charges of involuntary manslaughter (and practicing medicine without a license), a fact worth remembering before you embark on your own version of the Master Cleanse.

The Mayo Clinic advises eating a healthy diet based on fruits and vegetables, whole grains, and lean sources of protein as a better alternative, with longer-lasting benefits, than going on a detox diet.

Which isn't to say that fasting is all bad. Recent animal studies have demonstrated that intermittent fasting for short periods of time may slow aging, protect against stroke damage, and slow cognitive decline. But extended fasting is, and always has been, incredibly dangerous.

Just add cayenne pepper and you've got yourself a Master Cleanse.

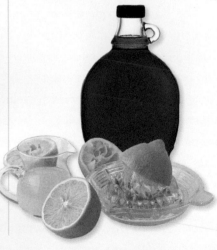

and was just the start of a prolific outpouring of writing in support of his ideas. Some of those—eating low fat, high-fiber foods, drinking lots of water, and getting outside—had merit. Other ideas, however, didn't.
From one of the brochures:

> Natural Hygiene rejects the use of medications, blood transfusions, radiation, dietary supplements, and any other means employed to treat or "cure" various ailments. These therapies interfere with or destroy vital processes and tissue. Recovery from disease takes place in spite of, and not because of, the drugging and "curing" practices.

The same brochure also described the Nature Cure approach to fasting:

> Fasting is the total abstinence from all liquid or solid foods except distilled water. During a fast the body's recuperative forces are marshaled and all of its energies are directed toward the recharging of the nervous system, the elimination of toxic accumulations, and the repair and rejuvenation of tissue. Stored within each organism's tissues are nutrient reserves which it will use to carry on metabolism and repair work. Until these reserves are depleted, no destruction of healthy tissue or "starvation" can occur.

Shelton obtained a substantial degree of popularity in the middle part of the twentieth century, operating a health school out of San Antonio, Texas, and running for president as part of the American Vegetarian Party (which took one-issue politics to a whole new level). He was also arrested, repeatedly for practicing medicine without a license. (And no, "Dr." Shelton, your physiological therapeutics degree doesn't count.)

In 1942, Shelton was charged with negligent homicide after a patient starved to death, but the case was dropped. Again, in 1978, Shelton was sued for negligence after another patient died at his school. This time he lost. The subsequent judgment bankrupted him and his health school closed, happily preventing any further lives from being lost.

But the quackery of the Natural Hygiene movement wasn't so easily defeated. After Shelton fell, a new trend rose to pick up the mantle of perverting the power of fresh air and sunshine. With supposedly ancient roots in Ayurvedic medicine, Breatharianism is the belief that human life can be exclusively sustained by cultivating *prana*, a universal life force found in all living things. Some Breatharians view sunlight as a primary generator of prana. Sunbathing, therefore, can be a substitute for eating . . . and drinking. Fun experiment: Try growing your houseplant without offering it any water. Watch what happens next.

Breatharianism found a foothold on the extremes of alternative health movements in the late twentieth century and was co-opted for monetary gain by charismatic charlatans like Wiley Brooks, founder of the Breatharian Institute of America, who first began espousing his crazy ideas on the TV show *That's Incredible!* in 1980. Brooks claimed to eat only when there was no fresh air to breathe, or when he couldn't get enough sunshine. He purported that humans, in their natural state, needed no other nourishment.

No other nourishment, that is, except for a Twinkie, a Slurpee, and a hot dog from 7-Eleven, all of which were seen clutched in Brooks's arms by an observer in 1983.

As his ideas devolved, Brooks began spewing some really out-there pseudo-philosophical mumbo-jumbo to justify his healthy diet of light, air, and junk food. Spiritually moved by the Double Quarter Pounder with Cheese at McDonald's, Brooks claimed that the burger possessed a special "base frequency" useful to Breatharians. You could wash it down with a Diet Coke because the soft drink made up of aspartame and dye is really "liquid light."

Confused yet? Not to worry, because somewhere between $100,000 and $1 billion will get you guidance from Brooks himself on how to live without food. In what must be an example of a Breatharian sliding scale, Brooks's Institute offers a payment plan to folks willing to fork up $10,000.

We could devote an entire book to cataloging charlatans like Brooks. And therein lies what makes this particular brand of quackery so dangerous: The problem with fasting, as opposed to say, neurosurgery, is that *anyone* can do it. Plenty of unqualified nonmedical professionals offer their opinions and advice. Even respectable writers get in on the game.

One of fasting's more enthusiastic adherents was none other than Upton Sinclair, author of *The Jungle* and famously gullible patient, who threw his full weight behind a variety of twentieth-century quack cures (see also Radionics, page 303). Sinclair's 1911 book, *The Fasting Cure*, detailed his personal experiments in not eating. Not content with merely describing his own experiences, Sinclair also offered general advice to the hundreds of people who wrote to him seeking his medical opinion—as a journalist— on whether fasting would help cure them. He recommended long fasts for those with "really desperate ailments" such as "Bright's disease, cirrhosis of the liver, rheumatism, and cancer." (Although modern doctors would strongly disagree with Sinclair's unsolicited medical advice, there have been some recent promising studies on the impact of fasting on mice with cancer. Human studies, however, are still lacking.)

In his book's preface, Sinclair recommends two places for fasting patients to "be taken charge of." In addition to Bernarr Macfadden's Healthatorium in Chicago, one other address is listed:

Dr. Linda B. Hazzard, of Seattle, Washington.

The Weight Loss Hall of Shame

Humans have long been on a tumultuous journey to fight gluttony and achieve an elusively perfect figure. What weapons we use in that battle change depending on the year and societal customs. The history of quackery is filled with weight-loss schemes that we have either tried ourselves or laughed at. Rub it away, purge it away, pop pills, eat only cabbage—these schemes have a past, present, and, no doubt, a future. So kick back, cheat on that cleanse with a cupcake, and enter the Weight Loss Hall of Shame.

TAPEWORMS

The tapeworm diet fad started in the 1800s. The idea is you eat tapeworm eggs, and the parasite eats your food for you. Often, the mail-order eggs were dead (or weren't there at all). A good thing, too, because an actual tapeworm infection might cause headaches, brain inflammation, seizures, and dementia. Tapeworms grow to thirty feet long, live for decades, and are hermaphrodites, which means they're making more tapeworms inside you. (Yep, you'd be hosting a tapeworm orgy!) So. Not. Worth. It.

SWEATING

In the nineteenth century, Charles Goodyear invented vulcanized rubber and voilà, the sado-masochist's version of Spanx was born in the form of rubber corsets and undies, promising to help sweat the fat away. Around the same time, other methods popped up, like vapor baths, dry heat, and light therapy (a sweltering 145°F treatment),

which offered a good weight loss–inducing sweat. But as any good wrestler or pounds-shedding MMA fighter will tell you, sweating as a means of weight loss is temporary. The weight returns, along with a pretty ravenous thirst.

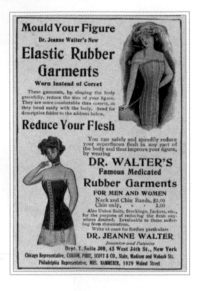

THYROID EXTRACTS

Boosting metabolism via thyroid extracts was very popular in the nineteenth and twentieth centuries. Since the thyroid gland helps regulate metabolism, dried and powdered glands from pigs and cows were found in nostrums like Dr. Newman's Obesity Pills. Sure, you might lose weight, but you could also get hyperthyroidism from all the excess hormones, giving you palpitations, sweating, bulging eyes, hair loss, and diarrhea.

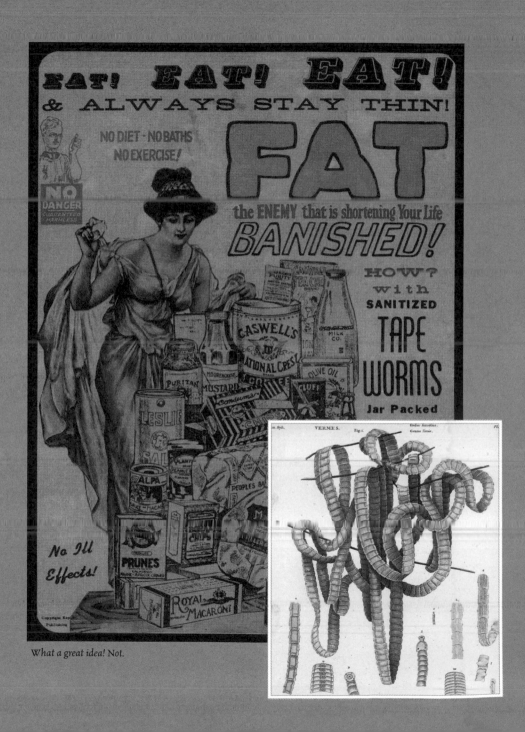

What a great idea! Not.

Because the element iodine is necessary to make thyroid hormone, some patent medicine pawners touted iodine-containing nostrums to boost metabolism. Did they work? Not really. Products like Allan's Anti-Fat contained bladderwrack, an iodine-rich seaweed found in many oceans. Nice idea, but products like this didn't budge your metabolism if your thyroid gland was already working fine.

DINITROPHENOL

A compound called dinitrophenol entered the market as a weight-loss medicine around 1934. Pro: It rapidly increased metabolism. Cons: It was used to create explosives, was carcinogenic, and had a nasty habit of killing people as they were "literally cooked to death" by the rapid increase in body temperature. The consolation prize wasn't great, either: If you didn't die, you might get a rash, loss of taste, and become blind. Yay! Because of the deaths and the terrible side effects, it disappeared off the market only four years later.

AMPHETAMINES

1-phenylpropan-2-amine, also known as amphetamine, Benzedrine, and Dexedrine, was synthesized in 1929. At first it was marketed for stuffy noses, then for minor depression. World War II servicemen received it to boost mood and alertness, but it had a surprising side effect of decreased appetite and weight loss. By the late 1960s, 4 billion doses (available without a prescription) were being manufactured per year.

The pills were also called "mother's little helpers" to create peppy, slim housewives. Unfortunately, they also caused "amphetamine psychosis," with users experiencing hallucinations (such as evil, talking toilet bowls) as they spiraled into addiction. In 1970, amphetamines finally came under tight restrictions, which probably quieted down a heckuva lot of talking toilets.

EXCESSIVE CHEWING

One diet fad wasn't about what you ate, but how many hundreds of times you chewed it. Horace Fletcher (d. 1914), called "The Great Masticator," promoted the excessive chewing of food to the point where it liquefied and became utterly tasteless. Any leftover fiber was spit out. If all went well with Fletcherism, you ate far less (too busy chewing) and you had a dismal social life. (Fletcher was reportedly a bore at meals because it's impolite to talk while chewing.) If you were a "super-masticator" you might have stools like Fletcher's—biscuitlike and so odorless you could parade them around and show them to people. Which is what Fletcher did.

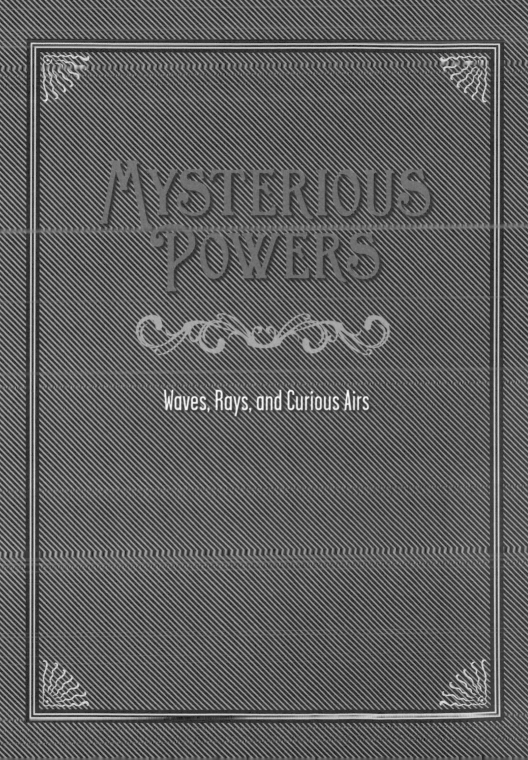

Mysterious Powers

Waves, Rays, and Curious Airs

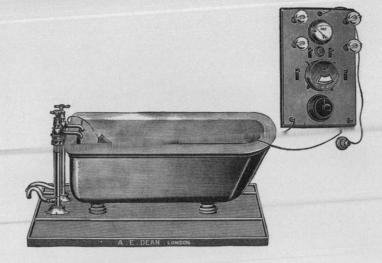

24

Electricity

Of Dancing Corpses, Electric Corsets,
the Pulvermacher, Galvanic Baths,
and the Eternal Beauty of Margaret Thatcher

On a cold January day in London in 1803, George Forster was hanged for the murder of his wife and child. In addition to hanging "until dead," Forster was sentenced to be dissected, a form of punishment that reached into the afterlife, for the general belief held that disassembled bodies could not be resurrected on Judgment Day. But Forster's body had another surprise on its way from gallows to grave: a public demonstration of the new scientific field of galvanism, that is, using electricity to stimulate muscles.

In the dark shadow of Newgate Prison, Forster's body was given to Giovanni Aldini, an Italian doctor with a taste for morbid theatrics, who propped Forster up in front of a crowd and ran electrical currents through the poor man's corpse.

The Newgate Calendar reported on what happened next:

> On the first application of the process to the face, the jaws of the deceased criminal began to quiver, and the adjoining muscles were horribly contorted, and one eye was actually opened. In the subsequent part of the process the right hand was raised and clenched, and the legs and thighs were set in motion.

The sight of Forster's newly hanged body, suddenly grimacing and flailing, caused such a sensation among the onlookers that many believed Forster had been resurrected from the dead. Genuine concern about this possibility

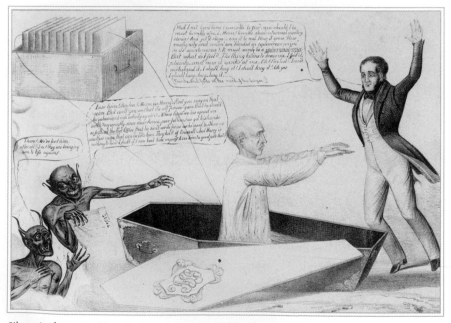

It's a miracle! Snatched from the demonic clutches of hell by the power of electricity!

was incorporated into his sentencing. In case the condemned man was indeed brought back to life by Aldini, the executioners were on standby, ready to promptly hang him again.

FROM LIGHTNING TO LABORATORY

The marvel and mystery of electricity has intrigued us since early humans were awestruck by the power of lightning. They also noticed that after amber was rubbed, it attracted hair and other light objects. They were witnessing what we today call the triboelectric effect, wherein materials acquire an electric charge after contact with something else. Most static electricity is triboelectric—the next time your clothes stick together after a bout in the dryer, you're witnessing the effect in action. It wasn't until 1600 that William Gilbert, part of Queen Elizabeth I's court, distinguished this reaction from magnetism (without the benefit of a clothes dryer) and coined the term *electricity* from the Greek *elektron*, for amber.

In the eighteenth century, scientific inquiry turned to electricity in earnest. The first Leyden jars were invented, solving the problem of how to store an electrical charge. And who could forget the image of Benjamin Franklin with his kite in Philadelphia's stormy sky in 1752? Franklin was followed by an Italian physicist, Alessandro Volta, who invented the first electric battery, and Luigi Galvani (Aldini's uncle) who discovered that the muscles of a dead frog's leg twitched when struck by an electric spark. That particular experiment involved hanging a bunch of dead frog legs on a metal banister during a storm. Galvani wasn't exactly a hit with his neighbors.

When Aldini provided the crowd at Newgate his gruesome and shockingly unethical spectacle with the corpse of George Forster, he was also demonstrating a very real, very important, and very new scientific breakthrough. For the first time in history, human beings could harness the power of electricity to manipulate the body.

In addition to stimulating frogs and criminal corpses, galvanism was embraced by medical practitioners aglow with the curative properties of electricity. A contemporary of Galvani, Christian Gottlieb Kratzenstein, began experimenting with medical uses of electricity by administering shocks to patients suffering from rheumatism, malignant fever, and the plague. Kratzenstein observed an increase in one's pulse after administering electrical shocks, which he believed aided the healing process in some diseases. He also observed that electrification of patients made them, somehow, tired. Kratzenstein suggested this effect might be beneficial for those whose "riches, sorrows, and worries prevent them from closing their eyes at night." Next time you can't sleep, just stick your finger into an outlet—just kidding, please don't do that.

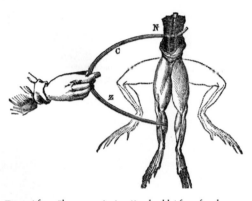

Excerpt from Ikea-esque instruction booklet for a frog leg electrocution kit.

In France, physicians began to experiment with electricity on paralyzed soldiers. On December 26, 1747, for example, a doctor drew sparks from a paralyzed arm for two hours in the morning and again for two to three hours in the afternoon. After enduring that treatment for a month (!), the patient was successfully cured of the paralysis. Other experiments were less conclusive, although the occasional success story and general excitement about the mysterious process of electrification led one French physician to comment "in this town, everybody wants to be electrified."

It wasn't long before quacks arose to fulfill that desire.

ELECTRIC BRUSHES,
CORSETS, AND BELTS

The public's enthusiasm for electricity was rampant in America as well, where a variety of devices were patented to help spread the electrical gospel, including electric brushes (for baldness!), electric corsets (for weight loss!), and electric belts (for erectile dysfunction!). Like the lines outside Apple stores whenever a new iPhone is released, people were practically tripping over themselves to acquire devices for self-electrification. New technology creates excitement, and excitement creates fertile ground for quackery.

In 1880, a certain Dr. Scott introduced an electric hairbrush, which quickly became all the rage in America. Dr. Scott's Electric Hair Brush contained a magnetized iron rod in its handle, but did not actually contain a, you know, *power source*. It was basically a mildly magnetized hairbrush, which is certainly a less sexy advertisement. But Scott, a genius at marketing, jumped on the electricity bandwagon, exploiting the little-understood phenomenon to make a tidy fortune.

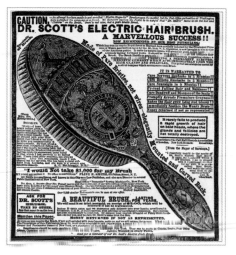

Scott, who plastered advertisements in newspapers across the country claimed that not only could his electric brush cure the

"A marvellous success!" "A beautiful brush!"

expected problems of baldness and headaches, but also—and the logic here falls flat on its face—such ailments as lameness, paralysis, and constipation.

Scott distributed his hairbrushes with a warning that simultaneously ensured higher sales and laid the groundwork for family squabbles: "In no case should more than one person use the brush. If always used by the same person it retains its full curative power."

Scott later expanded his non-electric electric empire to include corsets. Like his hairbrushes, Scott's "electric" corsets were just slightly magnetized. Advertised as "unbreak-able"—one shudders at the thought of forcing a human body into an "unbreakable" corset—the electric corsets could cure all manner of unlikely diseases. The corsets could also, when "constantly worn," become "equalizing agents in all cases of extreme fatness or leanness by

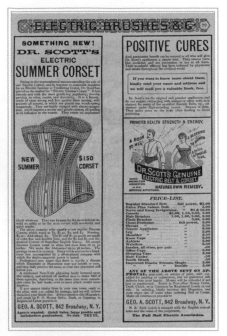

Cinch that waist with some electricity!

imparting the required amount of odic force which Nature's law demands."

Women weren't the only ones to benefit from the curative properties of electricity. Men were granted electric belts.

Enter the Pulvermacher.

If you were a fashionable, wealthy man in the late nineteenth century, you probably had a Pulvermacher. In addition to being an excellent name for a German death metal band, "Pulvermacher" was shorthand for the Pulvermacher Electric Belt, the crème-de-la-crème of electric belts at the turn of the century. The belts provided "mild, continuous currents" of electricity during the eight to twelve hours per day you were supposed to wear them. In addition to belts, the Pulvermacher Galvanic Company (headquartered at the Galvanic Establishment in San Francisco) produced a variety of electric chains that could be attached to almost any part of the body.

The zeal of electric belt wearers even made its way into fiction. In Gustave Flaubert's novel *Madame Bovary*, the character Homais is described as being "enthusiastic about the hydro-electric Pulvermacher chains; he wore one himself, and when at night he took off his flannel vest, Madame Homais stood quite dazzled before the golden spiral beneath which he was hidden, and felt her ardour redouble for this man more bandaged than a Scythian, and splendid as one of the Magi."

Pulvermacher belts, constructed with zinc and copper and soaked before use in vinegar, did in fact produce light currents of electricity by drawing out a minor current from the human body itself (so it was, quite accurately, "galvanic"). The current was just enough to ensure the wearer that the belt or chain was working.

This surety was also grounded in the aggressively confident promotional materials from the Pulvermacher Company, who made a habit of filling their "Electricity Is Life" advertisements with lengthy endorsements from prominent physicians. The only problem was they never actually attracted any endorsements, so they just made some up.

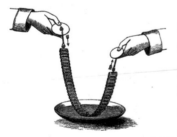

Electric belts were, of course, advertised as cure-alls, attacking ailments of the kidneys, stomach, liver, bowels, and, particularly, dyspepsia. Special models of electric belts also included a connection for the penis, which could be stimulated into action by the magic of galvanic current. Manufacturers played up a common fear of the late nineteenth century—that men had only a finite supply of semen they could distribute throughout their lifetime. Masturbation early in life, therefore, was blamed as the source of later problems with erectile dysfunction. Happily, running a light electric current into a tired old penis could go a long way to restoring it to its former glory days.

The delicate preparation of the electric belt.

Let's Mix Electricity with Water!

If you weren't getting the expected results from your corsets or belts, you could up the ante by soaking in an electric bath. Despite the generally sound principle of avoiding contact between water and electricity, a nineteenth-century movement led to the development of electric, or "galvanic," bathhouses. One such bathhouse—the Therapeutic and Electrical Institute—was opened by Jennie Kidd Trout, later commemorated on a Canadian stamp as the first woman to obtain a medical license in Canada. When Trout opened her institute in Toronto in 1875, it included six bathhouses. Patients would submerge a part or the entirety of their bodies in warm water in a metal-plated bathtub. The patients then held on to electrodes (not submerged, thankfully) connected to batteries, allowing a low-level current to electrify the water. It was basically a hot tub, but with the electricity inside the water rather than outside it.

It is worth noting that Trout, who also operated a free dispensary for the poor, was an intelligent, well-intentioned doctor and did not falsely advertise the medical claims from her treatments. She, along with many other physicians in the era, genuinely believed the electric bath treatments were helpful to her patients. The electric current was supposed to stimulate your organs and circulation, while the heat from the warm water also "opened your pores" and induced sweating to help flush out your toxins. As such, electric baths were advertised to help with a variety of chronic conditions such as rheumatism, gout, and sciatica.

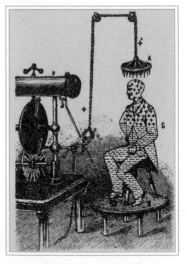

Although electric baths are no longer part of mainstream practice, they are still used in the medical underground. As

Russian electricity shower. Looks legit.

recently as 1989, a minor scandal broke out when *Vanity Fair* reported that the United Kingdom's Prime Minister Margaret Thatcher regularly took electric baths as part of an elaborate health and beauty routine. The prime minister visited a "certain Indian woman" who supposedly treated "the most high-powered women in the world." Thatcher paid upward of £600 for her special bath treatments, where 0.3 amps of electricity were run through the water.

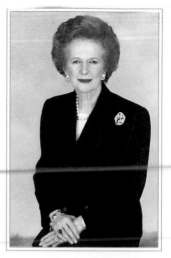

The "Switched-On Prime Minister."

The British tabloids had a field day with this news, with headlines like "Indian Guru Keeps Her Switched On—Maggie's Bathtime Secrets" and "The Switched-On Prime Minister's Amazing Secret."

Did the baths work? Well, you would hope so for £600 a treatment. Although there is no scientific causality at play here, Thatcher did attract endless tabloid speculation toward the end of her career about her ability to appear younger as she grew older. So it was either the electric baths or the natural vigor generated by crushing a welfare state and destroying worker pensions.

ELECTRICITY TODAY

Although electric baths, belts, and corsets have largely disappeared, the twentieth century produced a variety of legitimate electrical devices, including the EKG (electrocardiogram), which measures the electric activity of the heart. Electricity has also been used by orthopedists to help bones in their healing process and by cardiologists to regulate heartbeats with pacemakers. And then, of course, there is the defibrillator, which has saved countless lives over the years by sending a vital electrical shock to the heart.

So the medical community has made its peace with electricity. Still, one misses the trend-setting Pulvermacher. Just think of how, in those serious old photos of New York businessmen, somewhere beneath those stuffy clothes an electric belt was quietly humming.

It's a more pleasant thought, anyway, than dancing corpses beneath the gallows at Newgate Prison.

THE TEMPLE OF HEALTH

The powerful placebo effect generated from the invisible magic of electricity was well exploited by quacks, perhaps none as artfully as James Graham, a Scottish "doctor" who inspired wealthy patrons to back his crazy plans. One such venture was the Temple of Health and Hymen at the Adelphi in London in 1780. The experience included scantily clad goddesses reciting odes to Apollo and "the largest and most elegant

An expensive date night.

medico-electrical apparatus in the world." Here's the kicker: the machine was just there as a display piece; Graham didn't actually use it on patients. Instead, the machine added to the atmosphere by "gently pervading the whole system with a copious tide of that celestial fire, fully impregnated with the purest, most subtle, and balmiest parts of medicines, which . . . flow softly into the blood and nervous system, with the electric fluid, or restorative aetherial essences."

Graham also had a Celestial Bed available for couples struggling with fertility. The bed, twelve feet long by nine feet wide, was supported by forty pillars of colored glass and decorated with large crimson tassels. Perfumes were blown in via glass tubes; melodious music played in the distance. Beneath the bed there were magnetic lodestones— to provide the "celestial fire"—along with an electrically charged vacuum tube that occasionally would crackle and, apparently, contribute to the erotic atmosphere. Couples willing to pay £50 were allowed use of the bed and guaranteed "immediate conception" to boot.

Despite the scantily clad goddesses and the sheer awesomeness of Graham's audacity, the temple went bankrupt two years later.

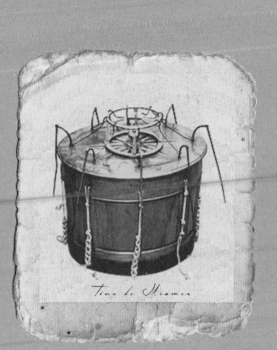

25

Animal Magnetism

Of Franz Mesmer, Father Hell, the Universal Magnetic Fluid, Grand Theatrics, and the Origins of Christian Science

Imagine you're a wealthy French noblewoman in 1788, suffering from those horrors of horrors: boredom and malaise. You've heard your friends talking about an exciting German physician and his strange new theories of animal magnetism. Indeed, you've heard of little else in the drawing rooms and parlors of Paris this past week. You decide to give this funny little man a try yourself, arriving at the delightfully well-appointed rooms at the House of Mesmer.

The light filters in through stained glass windows on the spacious saloon. All the walls are adorned with mirrors. The scent of orange blossoms wafts through the air. In the distance, you hear gentle singing and the light strumming of a harp.

In the center of the room, you see a large oval vessel, about four feet long and one foot deep. Inside, there are a large number of wine bottles, filled with "magnetized water." An assistant comes in and pours more water into the vessel, filling it to the top of the bottles. He then covers it with a hole-laden iron sheet called a baquet and inserts long rods into each opening. The other participants, almost all upper-class women like yourself, are invited to press the afflicted parts of their bodies—legs, arms, backs, and necks—against these iron rods to engage the healing powers of the magnetized water.

You are encouraged to sit close together around the baquet, with your legs touching your neighbor's, to "facilitate the passage of magnetic fluid."

Once everyone is in position, the "assistant magnetizers" appear and begin gently touching the knees, spines, and yes, even breasts of your fellow participants, all while staring directly into their eyes. They intend to manipulate the "universal fluid" within each of you through touch. The assistant magnetizers, you notice, are young and handsome. You are shocked and more than a little bit scandalized.

Some of your neighbors begin laughing hysterically, others begin sobbing, some shriek, some scream, some flee the room, and some faint. As for you, well, you certainly are feeling cured (for the moment) of your boredom and malaise.

Once the room has descended into mass delirium, you watch as the great prophet himself, Franz Mesmer, finally enters the parlor. An attractive man in his midforties, he is dressed in a long white robe embroidered with golden flowers. In his hands, he holds a large "magnetized" rod. Mesmer moves slowly from woman to woman gently stroking her with said rod to restore her to calmness again. You watch as one by one, your fellow patients relax.

By the time Mesmer approaches you, magnetic rod extended, you can take this scene no longer and you quickly flee the room. As you walk back into the afternoon light, you reflect that although it was perhaps the most ridiculous scene you have ever witnessed, you have to admit you were completely entertained. And you'll now have a shocking new topic of conversation at your next house party.

What just happened? To explain, we have to step a bit further back in time and introduce you to Father Hell.

FATHER HELL AND THE BIRTH OF ANIMAL MAGNETISM

In the 1770s, Franz Friedrich Anton Mesmer was a young doctor practicing medicine in Vienna, when a chance encounter with a Jesuit priest named Maximilian Hell changed his life forever. Maximilian Hell, or Father Hell, as we hope he preferred to be called, was conducting medical experiments with magnetized lodestone plates. Hell applied these plates to the naked bodies of sick patients in an effort to provide comfort for diseases like rheumatism.

Mesmer was enthralled by the priest's demonstrations. He adopted Hell's magnetic theory, and then twisted it into his own delightfully bizarre philosophy that all disease—literally every single disease—was the result of an imbalance in the body of a universal magnetic fluid that was susceptible to gravitational force. Mesmer initially believed that these imbalances could be redressed with the application of magnets, but soon became convinced that the true power to realign magnetic fluids lay within himself.

Calling this universal magnetic fluid "animal magnetism," Mesmer believed that by laying his hands on patients and engaging his willpower, he could manipulate this fluid and heal the sick.

The idea that human bodies contained a mysterious, universal fluid that could be influenced by external forces wasn't new and was, in fact, a basic tenet of occult movements such as astrology and alchemy. In the sixteenth century, Paracelsus suggested our systems could be affected by planetary movements. Mesmer built upon this theory in his dissertation at the University of Vienna in 1766, writing:

> The sun, moon, and fixed stars mutually affect each other in their
> orbits; that they cause and direct in our earth a flux and reflux
> not only in the sea, but in the atmosphere, and affect in a similar
> manner all organized bodies through the medium of a subtle and
> mobile fluid, which pervades the universe, and associates all things
> together in mutual intercourse and harmony.

Mesmer claimed that this "nervous fluid," or "animal magnetism" as he called it, could be manipulated by a physician. In an era of incredible new scientific discoveries such as electricity and gravity, Mesmer's magnetic fluid gospel found a willing audience.

Mesmer's Magic Touch

After convincing Father Hell to make some similar magnetic plates for him to experiment with, Mesmer started treating patients in Vienna. He met with early success while treating Franziska Oesterlin, a young "hysteric" suffering from convulsions. During an attack, Mesmer applied the magnetic plates to her stomach and legs. Oesterlin reported feeling "painful currents of a subtle material" traveling through her body, which reduced the severity of a convulsion, ultimately stopping it altogether.

He treated Oesterlin during many attacks over the next two years, eventually concluding that the magnetic plates were merely an accessory to Mesmer's touch itself. He found he could produce similar results by simply passing his hands along Oesterlin's body, or by moving his hands in the direction he wanted the magnetic fluid to travel, even from a great distance.

After declaring Oesterlin cured, Mesmer set about writing to all the learned societies of Europe about his exciting new discovery. It was a delightfully simple and bizarre theory: Human health depends upon the uninterrupted flow of animal magnetism throughout the body. If that magnetic fluid is blocked, disease is the inevitable result. Health could be restored by removing the block and manipulating the animal magnetism via a magnetized, well, *anything*.

Mesmer clarified this, sort of, while writing to a friend in Vienna:

I have observed that the magnetic is almost the same thing as the electric fluid, and that it may be propagated in the same manner, by means of intermediate bodies. Steel is not the only substance adapted to this purpose. I have rendered paper, bread, wool, silk, stones, leather, glass, wood, men, and dogs—in short, everything I touched—magnetic to such a degree that these substances produced the same effects as the loadstone on diseased persons.

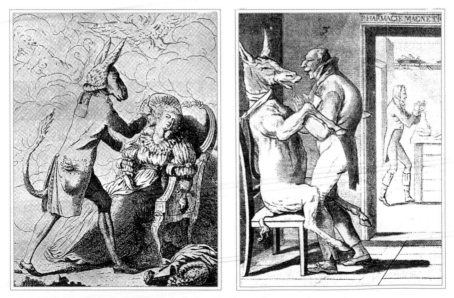

Of course, the satirists had a field day: here, donkeys hard at work as animal magnetizers.

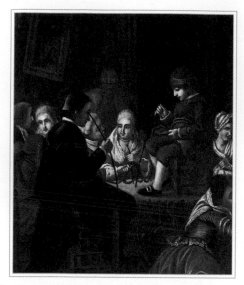

The nonstop action of facilitating the passage of magnetic fluid.

Taking a break from magnetizing leather and dogs, Mesmer landed a high-profile patient in Maria Theresia von Paradis, a young piano prodigy who had been blind since infancy. He attempted to adjust the young girl's animal magnetism and, apparently, even made some progress in curing her blindness before he was abruptly dismissed by the pianist's caregivers. Reports vary on the reason—some theorize that doctor and patient grew a little too close, which would hardly be a surprise considering all that intense touching going on—regardless, Mesmer was sent packing from Vienna.

THE SOCIETIES OF HARMONY

Despite the scandal back home in Austria, Mesmer found a more enlightened audience in France. His attractiveness, combined with his sophistication and almost preternatural self-confidence, found a natural sympathy with the French people. In 1778, he set up shop among the fashionable circles of Paris and launched his incredibly popular magnetic healing practice, which was two parts theater to one part healing. (Well, more like nine parts theater to one part healing.)

The drama and sexual undertones were perfect for the repressed audience. Mesmer's shows were an enormous hit and the physician was soon a wealthy man. Like so many quacks before and after him, as Mesmer's bank

AMERICAN INNOVATION: FROM MAGNETISM TO FAITH HEALING

In 1862, Mary Patterson was weak, emaciated, and depressed from spending much of her forty-two years sick and bedridden. Desperate for a cure, she limped her aching body up the stairs to the office of Phineas Parkhurst Quimby in Portland, Maine.

A few years earlier, Quimby had caught a lecture on animal magnetism from a visiting Frenchman named Charles Poyen. He was hooked. Like a 1990s teenager who caught his first Phish show and then gave up everything to follow the band around the country, Quimby resigned from his business and became a mesmerism groupie. He followed Poyen, learning everything he could.

Quimby's method of magnetic healing relied upon building rapport between physician and patient, encouraging them to improve their mental health through positive thinking. He would stare into his patients' eyes and listen carefully as they discussed their health complaints while he massaged their hands and arms. Somehow, Quimby was not viewed as creepy. Quite the opposite; after simply being listened to by their physician, a lot of Quimby's patients were subsequently "cured."

Quimby appears to have been a genuine believer in the mesmeric healing arts he practiced. Although Mesmer's morals were swallowed up in his mad dash for money and celebrity, Quimby had faith in the procedure and tried to help as many sick people as he could.

Including the poor young woman who stepped into his office that day in 1862.

To everyone's shock, including her own, after just a week with Quimby staring intensely into her eyes and massaging her hands, Patterson reported a sudden and dramatic improvement in her health. Soon Quimby had more than a patient on his hands: He had a die-hard devotee.

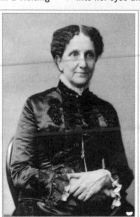

Mary Baker Eddy (née Patterson).

The newly energized Patterson learned everything she could from Quimby before developing her own medical system influenced by animal magnetism. She later got married and adopted the name history would remember her by. Mary Baker Eddy. Oh, and that little medical system she invented? It was the beginning of Christian Science, the largest healing faith ever produced in America, still going strong in 2017 with a global membership of about four hundred thousand people.

Mary modified the magnetic healing theories of Quimby and Mesmer to add a religious element: All disease is an illusion that can be cured by communion with God. And so animal magnetism continues—albeit in a modified form—into the twenty-first century.

account grew, his moral commitments to advancing medicine shrank. And then they shrank some more.

Mesmer never lacked audacity, however, and he soon wrote the queen, Marie Antoinette herself, asking for a château and a significant annual income from the royal coffers for, well, basically just being Mesmer:

> In the eyes of your majesty, four or five hundred thousand francs, applied to a good purpose, are of no account. The welfare and happiness of your people are everything. My discovery ought to be received and rewarded with a munificence worthy of the monarch to whom I shall attach myself.

The queen's advisers eventually replied, offering a 20,000-franc pension if Mesmer could prove his discovery successfully in front of physicians appointed by the king. Mesmer demurred and, suddenly proclaiming his disdain for money, fled Paris (and with it, the possibility of further investigation) for the Belgian town of Spa. Some enthusiastic converts followed, where one of them, named Bergasse, opened a subscription service in his

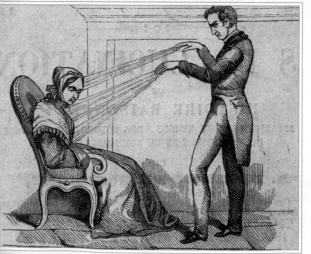

name. Each subscriber, at the rate of one hundred louis d'or each, would receive their leader's secrets. Mesmer, forgetting his earlier disdain for money, happily agreed, receiving a fortune of 140,000 francs from subscribers who wanted to spread the Mesmerian gospel.

Money in hand, Mesmer triumphantly returned to Paris, while his subscribers opened what they called Societies of

A life-size puppet (from a French magnetism manual, 1846).

Harmony throughout France, where they purported to cure disease through magnetism. It was no accident that many of the subscribers were wealthy libertines, eager to set up magnetized healing rituals for the debauched pleasure of watching young women descend into delirious states.

Mesmer's return to Paris, however, did not escape the notice of the comparatively austere French Academy of Sciences, who decided to look into this sweeping medicinal trend in 1784. They even roped visiting American dignitary Benjamin Franklin into their investigation. Their bummer of a conclusion: Magnetic fluid did not exist. Mesmer was decried as a fraud, using the powers of suggestion and imagination to create powerful placebo effects in his patients.

Mesmer left France for good and drifted into obscurity, wandering around Europe before dying in Austria in 1815. His legacy, however, lives on. Today, Merriam-Webster defines *mesmerize* as to "hypnotize" or "spellbind."

But magnetism wasn't done. Mesmer actually laid the groundwork for a surprisingly effective form of relaxation and pain relief. How? To explain, we must journey to Bengal, India, where a doctor was dealing with a rather *large* problem.

HYPNOSIS:
MAGNETISM'S MODERN UPGRADE

James Esdaile was a British colonial doctor serving in Bengal who was anxious to provide pain relief for his patients while he attempted to drain their large scrotal tumors. A result of an outbreak of filariasis, a parasitic disease from roundworm infections, the problem was of such a massive scale (one man's scrotal tumor was so large that he had to move it via a rope and pulley system) that the medical community was struggling to provide a solution.

Although this was thousands of miles away from Paris, word had trickled down to the remote outposts of the colonial empire of a certain Franz

Mesmer who was producing trance states in patients that allowed for pain-free medical procedures.

Esdaile read up on Mesmer, then decided to give animal magnetism a go himself. The doctor improvised a unique mesmeric method that included elements of local Indian practice, such as yogic breathing and stroking. After the patient slipped into a trance state, out came the scalpel, and—hopefully—out came the scrotal tumor. The funny thing was, it worked.

Although Esdaile would have considered himself a Mesmerist (the term *hypnosis* was just then coming into use in England), he effectively pioneered the use of hypnosis for surgical anesthesia, which would flourish briefly prior to the discovery of chloroform and was used effectively all the way through the American Civil War. In an era when on a good day a surgeon would manage to *not* kill 50 percent of his patients, Esdaile lost only sixteen patients out of the thousands he operated on during his six years in India.

The use of hypnotism in Western medicine really took off, however, when Scottish surgeon James Braid managed to elevate hypnotic techniques into mainstream medical practice. Like many physicians of his day, Braid was introduced to hypnotic techniques via a public demonstration of animal magnetism, which he first witnessed in 1841. Braid was amazed at what he saw and returned the following week to watch the same demonstration again. Convinced that he had observed a unique phenomenon, but dissatisfied with its explanations of manipulated "emanations" or "magnetic fluids," Braid sought his own answers.

During both demonstrations of animal magnetism, Braid noticed that the patient's eyes had remained closed. He concluded that the patient had somehow been lulled into sleep due to neuromuscular exhaustion, probably induced via intense staring. He decided to experiment on his dinner guest the next evening, whom he invited to stare without blinking at the top of a wine bottle for as long as possible. The dinner guest promptly fell asleep (and never went back for another dinner at Braid's house).

After repeating the experiment to similar success with his wife and man-servant, Braid enjoyed having the house to himself for a few minutes, put his feet up on the dinner table without anyone yelling at him, and reached an important conclusion: The mesmerized state, which he would dub "nervous sleep," could be understood as a physiological and psychological phenomenon.

Braid spent the next eighteen years of his life researching hypnosis and employing it in a wide variety of medical applications, including the treatment of spinal curvature, deafness, and epilepsy. He claimed his treatments worked, and they were gradually accepted by the medical community owing to Braid's investigations and near-constant stream of publications in academic journals. The physician laid the groundwork for the occasional accepted medical use of hypnosis, which includes treatment for pain, hot flashes, fatigue, and many psychological ailments.

Braid was even responsible for popularizing the name that history would remember the practice by: hypnosis. It's thanks to Braid that today you seek out treatment from a hypnotherapist and not an "animal magnetizer."

Isn't that something to be thankful for?

26

Light

Of Blue Glass, Kellogg's Light Baths, the Spectro-Chrome Institute, the Surgical Ray, and the Bureau of Cosmotherapy

Brigadier General Augustus J. Pleasanton was a respectable citizen of mid-nineteenth-century Philadelphia who happened to spend an inordinate amount of time puzzling over the sky. "For a long time I have thought that the blue color of the sky, so permanent and all-pervading . . . must have some abiding relation and intimate connection with the living organisms on this planet."

Pleasanton decided to experiment with this idea and got to work constructing a greenhouse with alternating blue panels on his estate in 1860, filling it with grapevines. His plants grew at an astonishing rate, although this was probably due to the fact that he built them a *greenhouse* and had nothing to do with the blue glass panels. Pleasanton was encouraged, however, and his grapes were the envy of his neighbors.

Then, in 1869, Pleasanton was staring at a pig one day and thought to himself, *What if I shone blue light on a pig?* So the intrepid inventor let some of his piglets develop in a piggery with clear glass and some in a piggery with blue glass. And, lo and behold, the blue light pigs grew quicker and were healthier.

This was all the confirmation Pleasanton needed. He was ready to loudly proclaim the gospel of blue light to anybody willing to listen. He soon landed on a charming, if entirely kooky, vision of the future of the human race where, thanks to harnessing the power of blue light, we become giants in perfect health, bringing along our domesticated animals for the ride:

> What strength of vitality could be infused into the feeble young,
> the mature invalid, and the decrepit octogenarian! How rapidly
> might the various races of our domestic animals be multiplied, and
> how much might their individual portions be enlarged!

His enthusiasm was contagious. As Pleasanton spread his views around the country in self-published pamphlets, reports began to trickle, then pour in, of illnesses cured and injuries alleviated by soaking up the rays beneath blue glass windowpanes.

Pleasanton even received a letter announcing that a premature baby, born paralyzed, had been placed beneath blue glass for long periods and was now able to move. Another attested to an infant whose large tumor had disappeared after exposing it for an hour each day to blue light. And so on.

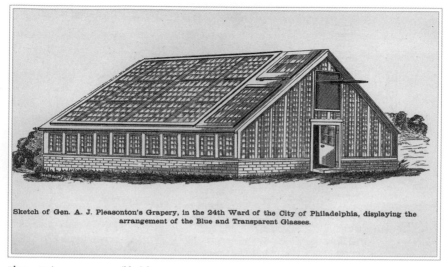

Sketch of Gen. A. J. Pleasonton's Grapery, in the 24th Ward of the City of Philadelphia, displaying the arrangement of the Blue and Transparent Glasses.

Pleasanton's awesome green (blue) house.

Pleasanton wrote a book about his blue light discoveries, chock full of such testimonials from patients, and, in an extraordinary effort to fill some blank pages, his own bizarre theories on electricity and electromagnetism. The coolest thing about Pleasanton's book, however, and the reason it's a collector's item today, is that he had it printed on blue paper with blue ink "to relieve the eyes of the reader from the great glare, occasioned by the reflection of gas light at night from the white paper usually employed in the printing of books." It was a thoughtful gesture to his readers, but an unfortunate choice for latter-day scholars who now must struggle to read the fading light blue ink.

Published in 1876, *The Influence of the Blue Ray of the Sunlight and of the Blue Colour of the Sky* launched the blue light fad into the mainstream for two glowing years. The second edition of Pleasanton's book, which claimed that blue glass was a universal panacea and could cure everything from gout to paralysis, came out the next year, and glass manufacturers around the country lined up in droves to personally thank the author.

From New York City to San Francisco, homeowners began adding sunrooms built with blue glass or, at the very least, a few blue windowpanes here and there. Hydropathic institutes also caved to public demand for blue light and began constructing blue light sunrooms. The trend soon spread to Europe, where "light baths" became very popular in England, and French opticians began to manufacture blue eyeglasses. In 1877, a journalist for *Scientific American* wrote:

> It is now quite common along our streets and avenues to see frames
> of azure crystals hanging within dwelling house windows; while,
> on sunny days, the invalid grandfather or other patient may be
> noticed basking in the ethereal rays, his countenance filled with
> hope, though streaked with blue.

That same article, however, was also the beginning of the end for the blue light fad. It was the first in a series produced by the magazine debunking the craze for being exactly—and only—that: a craze. *Scientific American* came out punching, announcing the scientific reality that lounging underneath blue glass actually exposed you to *less* blue light, not more. If you really wanted to soak up blue rays, you were better off standing outside or, at the very least, beneath clear glass. Really all Pleasanton had been doing—and all that anyone else had been doing, for that matter—was slightly shading sunlight. A week after that damning piece, *Scientific American* struck again, proclaiming that the supposed cures generated by blue light were a combination of the well-studied health benefits of a brief sunbath and a pronounced placebo effect.

Despite attempted rebuttals from Pleasanton, the end was nigh. By 1878, the general public had moved on, and the blue glass craze faded away just as quickly as it had sprung up. Although the obsession with blue light had died down, the process of using light to heal did not disappear as quickly. Medical quacks of the late nineteenth and early twentieth centuries continued with variations on a general "light as healer" theme.

ARTIFICIAL SUN: LIGHT THERAPY
MOVES INDOORS

In 1879, Thomas Edison first demonstrated his version of the incandescent lightbulb. Although Edison was not the first person to invent a lightbulb, he was the first to invent one that was commercially viable, could be produced cheaply, and had a long lifetime—twelve hundred hours. Edison didn't stop there. He went on to develop an electrical grid system, demonstrating how electricity could enlighten an entire community from a central generator wired to each home. He even created the first electric meter to measure use. By the time he was done, Edison said, "We will make electricity so cheap that only the rich will burn candles."

Edison's groundbreaking work paved the way for physicians to experiment with the impact of concentrated light on disease. Some legitimate uses of light therapy were subsequently developed, particularly by Niels Ryberg Finsen, who won the Nobel Prize in Medicine in 1903 for demonstrating the susceptibility of lupus to concentrated light radiation.

But quacks were quick to get in on the action, too.

In the late 1890s, John Harvey Kellogg invented "light baths" (in addition to breakfast cereal) for use at his sanitarium in Battle Creek, Michigan. From an 1893 newspaper article:

> The necessary parts are a cabinet that encloses the entire body except the head, and fifty electric lamps of sixteen-candle power or 110 volts. They are arranged about the body in groups, with a separate switch for each group, so they can be directed at a particular part of the body. The light makes the patient frisky, and browns the skin like an ocean bath.

Basically, using the bath was like sitting in a sauna with really harsh lighting. Kellogg believed that light baths could cure typhoid, scarlet fever, and diabetes,

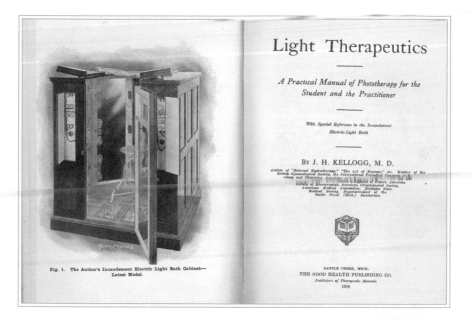

Fig. 1. The Author's Incandescent Electric Light Bath Cabinet—
Latest Model.

Light Therapeutics

*A Practical Manual of Phototherapy for the
Student and the Practitioner*

With Special Reference to the Incandescent
Electric-Light Bath

By J. H. KELLOGG, M. D.

Author of "Rational Hydrotherapy," "The Art of Massage," etc. Member of the
British Gynæcological Society, the International Periodical Congress
rology and Obstetrics, Medical Society of France, American
Society of Microscopists, American Climatological Society,
American Medical Association, Michigan State
Medical Society, Superintendent of the
Battle Creek (Mich.) Sanitarium

BATTLE CREEK, MICH.
THE GOOD HEALTH PUBLISHING CO.
Publishers of Therapeutic Manuals
1910

"Very short applications over the heart are useful in cases of collapse under anesthesia, opium poisoning, and in cases of heart failure." (From Light Therapeutics' section on shining an arc light over your chest.)

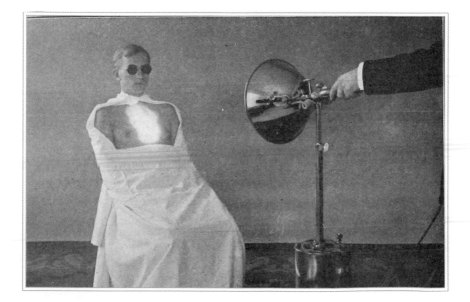

and could help treat obesity, scurvy, and constipation. In 1910's *Light Therapeutics: A Practical Manual of Phototherapy for the Student and the Practitioner*, he wrote of the benefits of the light bath:

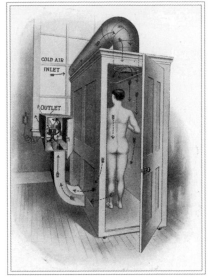

Nudity allowed in the light box.

> The electric-light bath prolonged to the extent of producing vigorous perspiration should be employed two or three times a week. . . . Tanning the whole surface of the body by means of the arc light will be an excellent means of improving the patient's general vital condition.

In other words, Kellogg stumbled upon the health benefits of sweating. He claimed that his light baths had been adopted by several of the "crowned heads and titled families of Europe" after King Edward of England was apparently cured of his gout by taking a series of light baths in Hamburg. Edward, we are assured by Kellogg, subsequently had a light bath installed at Windsor and Buckingham. So now you've got your question for the tour guide next time you visit either palace.

No Diagnosis, No Drugs, No Problem?

Dinshah P. Ghadiali was a stage manager in Bombay, India, when he first read about color therapy. Inspired, he leapt to the aid of a friend's niece—who was suffering from mucous colitis—with nothing more than a purple pickle bottle, a kerosene lamp, and some milk in a blue glass container. After she was "cured," Ghadiali knew he'd found his calling and emigrated to the United States in 1911 to spread the color-therapy gospel—and make a pretty penny while he was at it.

Ghadiali blended elements of lightbulb therapy and the blue glass trend to create what he called the Spectro-Chromo Institute. For a $100 cash advance, you could enroll in his intensive courses in spectro-chromo therapy and learn all about the "restoration of the human Radio-Active and Radio-Emanative Equilibrium by Attuned Color Waves" from Ghadiali himself—who, we are assured, was such an innate genius that back in his native India he was teaching college courses in mathematics when he was but a wee lad of eleven. (Ghadiali was so enamored of himself that he added this behemoth to his signature line: "M.D., M.E., D.C., Ph.D., L.L.D., N.D., D. Opt., D.F.C., D.H.T., D.M.T., Etc.")

The basic premise of his therapy was that every element exhibits one of the seven prismatic colors. Human beings are made up mostly of oxygen, hydrogen, nitrogen, and carbon, which in turn correspond to blue, red, green, and yellow. Feeling a bit ill? One of your colors is out of whack. To cure a disease, you just needed to have your faded colors amplified or your overly brilliant colors toned down.

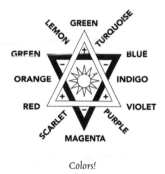

Colors!

To perform this action, Ghadiali invented a device called a Spectro-Chrome, which was basically a box with a 1,000-watt lightbulb inside it (see page 292 for a photo). Users could place colored glass plates in a window in the box to soak up the rays of specifically colored light. (Just like the blue glass craze, however, by shading the light the user was actually absorbing *less* of their chosen color.) Like a kinky version of an Easy-Bake Oven, the Spectro-Chrome required standing—nude—in front of the light box during specific lunar phases. The impact of the moon cycle on an electrically operated light box remains . . . mysterious.

THE SURGICAL RAY AND THE BUREAU OF COSMOTHERAPY

Around the same time that Ghadiali was transporting his secretary across state lines, colored glass made a comeback when the Von Schilling Surgical Ray hit the market. Basically a thick circle of colored glass similar to a hand mirror, the Surgical Ray could be held above your ache or injury to concentrate a particular color of light on it.

Following similar principles, the book *The Seven Keys to Colour Healing: A Complete Outline of the Practice* was written by Roland Hunt of the Bureau of Cosmotherapy (haven't you heard of it?) in 1940. Hunt used bad poetry as a way to underscore his points about the benefits of chromotherapy:

In Coolness new, as refreshing dew
Tone Thou my speech, O Ray of Blue—
And make It True,
And make It True.

The claim for which Hunt was so desperately seeking veracity was the notion that blue-tinted water—which he dubbed "Ceruleo"—could cure dysentery, cholera, and the bubonic plague. By way of evidence, Hunt assured his readers (assuming there was more than one) that in Bombay thousands of lives had been saved from the plague by the consumption of Ceruleo.

Not sure which color to use for your particular injury or disease? No worries—the Spectro-Chrome came with a special chart to help you navigate this complex decision-making process. Yellow light aided food digestion, green light stimulated pituitary glands, red light built hemoglobin, blue light increased vitality, lemon light restored bones. And so on.

Somehow, the Spectro-Chrome was a hit: Ghadiali had sold nearly eleven thousand devices by 1946, earning over one million dollars. Like Kellogg, who touted noninvasive, non-pharmaceutical procedures, Ghadiali's promise of "No Diagnosis, No Drugs, No Surgery" struck a chord with an audience that was wary of the medical establishment. And the medical establishment wasn't happy about that.

In 1925, the successful salesman was arrested after transporting his nineteen-year-old secretary across state lines for "immoral purposes." It wasn't

THE VIOLET RAY

At the intersection of electrotherapy and light therapy was the violet ray, invented by Nikola Tesla and first demonstrated at the World's Columbian Exposition in 1893. The device applied a high voltage and high frequency (but low current) stream of electricity to the body as a healing agent. When the glass electrode was energized, it emitted an intriguing and mysterious violet glow, which in and of itself produced a powerful placebo effect (because, cool!). The devices were manufactured by a variety of US companies and advertised for numerous conditions, including "brain fog," which could be cured by the following method:

> Applicator No. 1 over forehead and eyes. Also treat the back of head and neck with a strong current in direct contact with the skin. Treat the spine and hold the electrode in the hand. Ozone inhalations for about four minutes are also of importance.

After numerous lawsuits and the intervention of the FDA, violet ray manufacturers were eventually forced to halt production in the early 1950s. Today, violet ray machines are a much sought-after item on the collector's market for their association with Nikola Tesla, who has obtained cultlike status in the years since his death, and because it is indeed pretty cool to see the violet ray light up a deep purple color. Meanwhile, a new device dubbed the "violet wand," which does basically the same thing as the violet ray but for a completely different reason, has been adopted by the BDSM community.

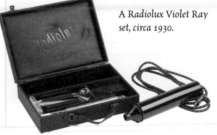

A *Radiolux Violet Ray* set, *circa* 1930.

his first—or last—brush with the law. Under intense scrutiny from the AMA and the FDA, Ghadiali had legal troubles for the rest of his life; his agile mind, however, always found new ways to sell his products. Instead of advertising its ability to "cure," Ghadiali's promotional material now advertised the "normalating" influence of the Spectro-Chrome. Patients were not being "treated," they were having their "radio-active and radio-emanative equilibrium" restored.

Once the language was switched, it was increasingly difficult for governmental authorities to prosecute Ghadiali for making false or misleading claims. If people really wanted to throw away their money on the "normalating influence" of a Spectro-Chrome machine, well, it's a free country.

Ghadiali died in 1966; his ideas have somehow survived him. The Dinshah Health Society of Malaga, New Jersey, a registered nonprofit administered by Ghadiali's heirs, is still in operation today selling a variety of light-therapy books and related products.

LIGHTING THE WAY FORWARD

Today, we know that light helps the body synthesize Vitamin D, and light therapy is used by modern physicians for the treatment of an assortment of ailments, including seasonal affective disorder, depression, jet lag, psoriasis, and infantile jaundice.

The real benefit that came out of the nineteenth century's blue light craze was really quite simple: the invention of the modern sunroom. Because it turns out that humans actually do enjoy the chance to sit around and soak up rays in the comfort of their own homes.

They just don't need blue windowpanes to do it.

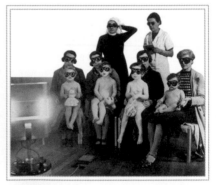

Children, with nurses, receive "ray treatment" in London, 1938.

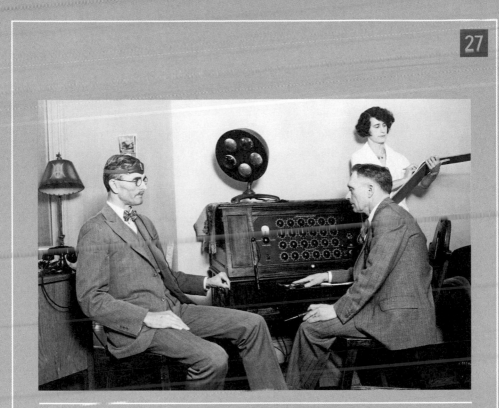

27

Radionics

Of Nickelback, the Dynamizer, the Oscilloclast, an "Eager and Excitable Little Jewish Doctor," an Undercover Guinea Pig, and Long-Distance Healing

Radio frequencies are difficult to understand. As with electricity and wi-fi, most of us are content just to know that radio waves work and are not concerned with *how* they work. You turn on the radio, dial into a station, and, like magic, you're suddenly listening to a song. And that song might possibly be *More Than a Feeling*, by Boston, one of the most frequently played radio songs of all time. There's something comforting in that.

In the early twentieth century, radio was the flashy new tech and had all the glamour and speculation about it that today surrounds driverless cars or even new iPhones. Thanks to recent technological advances by Italian inventor Guglielmo Marconi, who created the first commercially successful radio transmission system in 1895, the popular excitement about radio waves, coupled with the lack of understanding about exactly how they worked, made a market ripe for exploitation. Medical cures that purported to harness this mysterious energy found a willing audience. This is why men like Dr. Albert Abrams were able to make a fortune by claiming to diagnose and treat illnesses . . . with radio waves.

BAD VIBES AND THE MAN TO CURE THEM

Born in San Francisco in 1863, Albert Abrams obtained his MD in Germany at the remarkably young age of nineteen and returned to his native city in 1893 to serve as a professor of pathology at Cooper College. By the time he was in his forties, Abrams had built a solid reputation as a neurologist and was well on his way toward a distinguished career. The cracks, however, were beginning to show.

After losing his professorship due to a night-class scam, Abrams leaned more and more toward quackery, developing questionable techniques like hammering along the spine (spondylotherapy) to stimulate nerves that, in turn, were thought to stimulate the organs and heal sicknesses. The practice was touted as a cure-all for anything that ailed you.

His star treatment, though, was radionics. In 1916, Abrams published *New Concepts in Diagnosis and Treatment*, introducing the world to his theories. And just what were those theories? The short version: Healthy people radiate healthy energy. Diseased people radiate illness frequencies, which radionics practitioners like Abrams claimed they could detect with complex, cumbersome machines. They could then cure your disease—*any* disease, by the way— by tuning your illness frequency back to a healthy frequency.

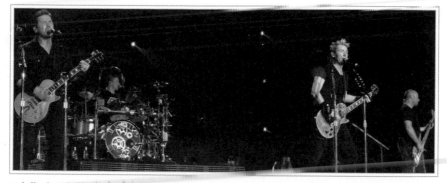

Nickelback probably playing "Photograph."

It's kind of like scanning the radio while you're on a road trip. By some terrible twist of fate, you might find yourself suddenly tuned to a Nickelback song. This is similar to the body emanating a diseased frequency. Luckily, it's just as easily fixed. Just like you can quickly turn the radio dial again, shuddering as you leave Nickelback safely behind you, a radionics practitioner with the right machine can just as easily retune your body to a healthy frequency.

Now for the long version (and please, pause here to take a deep breath): The human body is made up of atoms; atoms in turn are made up of electrons. Electrons vibrate, transmitting radiation, identified by radionics professionals as "ERA," or "electronic reactions of Abrams." If an individual is healthy, his or her electrons vibrate at a "normal" rate. If an individual is unhealthy, however, that person's electrons vibrate at an "abnormal" rate. So, to cure a patient, a physician had to detect the unhealthy vibrations, then transmit back at the disease the same vibratory frequency that the diseased electrons were producing. This would in turn neutralize the disease and allow the electrons to return to normal vibration rates.

Returning to our Nickelback scenario, it's like trying to get rid of one of their songs by aiming your iPod at the radio speakers, cuing up Nickelback, and blasting it back.

And it works just about as well.

DIAGNOSING WITH THE DYNAMIZER

So, how did radionics practitioners detect the abnormal vibrations? In predictably absurd ways.

Let's say you just received a bummer of a diagnosis from your conventional doctor. As a coping mechanism, you remind yourself that it's always worthwhile to get a second opinion and, hey, this Dr. Abrams you've heard about is supposed to be able to cure anything. Why not give him a try?

After a call to his office, you are instructed to bring in a hair sample. Scratching your head at the logic there, you pluck out a hair and make your way to Abrams's San Francisco establishment.

When you arrive, the receptionist asks if you collected your hair sample while you were facing west. She insists that this is a crucial element of the diagnosis. You don't remember which way you were facing, so, reluctantly, you face the setting sun and again pluck a few hairs from your head.

Satisfied finally, the receptionist brings you into Abrams's office and directs you to place your hair sample in a strange-looking medical machine she calls a Dynamizer. Enter Dr. Abrams, a confident man who bustles around the room, dimming the lights and hooking you up to the Dynamizer with a variety of wires that, he assures you, will detect your "vibrational patterns." You are once again instructed to face west because this will ensure the proper functioning of the machine.

Abrams then hooks up the Dynamizer to a series of other machines, including one he calls a Radioclast; its defining feature, you decide, is that it simply has a lot of dials on it. The doctor assures you that the dials will be greatly useful in detecting "ohmage," which will in turn help him pinpoint your exact disease.

He then instructs you to unbutton your shirt and pull up your undershirt. While you do so, Abrams retrieves a glass rod from his desk and begins to gently stroke your abdomen with it. You ask what exactly he hopes

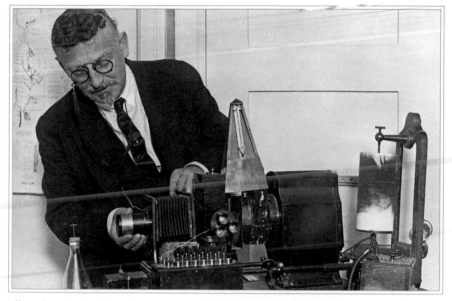

Albert Abrams looking like a doctor as he manipulates a totally bullshit machine.

to gain from this. The doctor says he is looking for areas of "resonance" or "dullness."

It all sounds very impressive, and you think to yourself that really, if he is going to all this fuss about "resonance" and "ohmage," then surely it must work. Right?

Too busy to make it into Abrams's office? No worries. Eventually, as radionics progressed, the patient's presence was not even necessary, and a skilled practitioner could detect the illness just by running the hair or blood (or handwriting) sample through the Dynamizer.

The electronic reactions were notoriously fickle. When collecting a sample, a patient had to face west, of course, and be in dim lighting, without any orange- or red-colored material in the room. Conveniently, the presence of skeptical minds could also drive away the vibrational reactions.

Radionics could not only supposedly detect disease, but it could also determine a person's sex, pregnancy stage, age, geographic location, and, of all things, the person's religion. Abrams even had a chart printed in 1922 that showed the abdominal areas of dullness for the various Christian denominations.

What's more, Abrams claimed to be able to use a handwriting sample from a dead person to identify what caused his or her demise. The Dynamizer was turned on the signatures of Samuel Pepys (syphilis), Dr. Samuel Johnson (syphilis), Henry Wadsworth Longfellow (syphilis), Oscar Wilde (syphilis), and Edgar Allan Poe ("the common cold"—just kidding, "syphilis and a reaction of dipsomania").

The Dynamizer was ready and willing to boldly declare that many of literary history's luminaries died of sexually transmitted disease. If you're shaking your head in total befuddlement, we don't blame you. Don't worry, though, because home courses in radionics were available for $200 cash, paid in advance.

The Lie of a Cure and the Rise of a Cult

Okay, so you've got your diagnosis now, courtesy of the Dynamizer, and because it was the Dynamizer, you probably just found out that you have syphilis. What to do next? Enter the Oscilloclast, the name for the radionics machine that could cure your ills (and should also be the name of someone on WrestleMania). To cure your syphilis, you would need to lease an Oscilloclast from Abrams, for an initial payment of either $200 or $250 (it was higher if wired for direct current, rather than alternating), plus $5 per month in perpetuity. Eventually, the doctor was netting $1,500 per month from leasing fees paid to him by lesser quacks.

Oscilloclast machines claimed to operate by directing radio waves at the patient. These radio waves were tuned to specific frequencies that would apparently kill off the infection or disease. "Specific drugs must have the same vibratory rate as the diseases against which they are effective," said

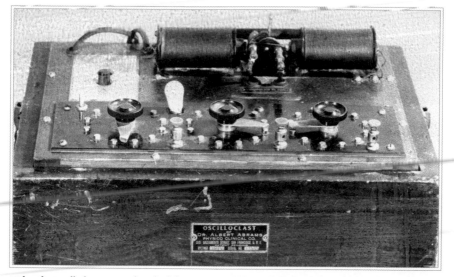

Either the Oscilloclast or a machine built by a ten-year-old boy to fool an eight-year-old boy.

Abrams. "That is why they cure." Or so the doctor believed. By extension, Oscilloclast machines could be tuned to the same "vibratory rate," that is, radio frequency, to cure disease as well.

Leased Oscilloclasts, however, had a particular condition, which the lessee had to agree to. You could not open the machine, which was "hermetically sealed." Opening the device would disrupt its functioning (and totally void that awesome Oscilloclast warranty).

The real reason you couldn't open the machine was that it contained nothing but a jumble of electrical parts wired together to no particular purpose. It was "the kind of device a ten-year-old boy would build to fool an eight-year-old boy," wrote a physicist after breaking the sacred radionics oath.

That consumers were essentially playing with toys didn't matter. Abrams struck gold with both the Oscilloclast and the Dynamizer. Their popularity largely stemmed from a simple psychological trick that was artfully exploited by Abrams and his followers: convince a person, through a quasi-religious medical ritual, that he has a disease such as cancer.

Then offer to cure the person with the Oscilloclast. Soon, the patient is happily free of cancer, a disease he never had in the first place. The patient can then spread the word among his friends. "I was so close to dying, you wouldn't believe it. But, thankfully, I heard about this new cure called radionics. They hooked me up to a machine, and *poof*, my cancer was gone!" That's powerful stuff and quickly builds a word-of-mouth marketing campaign.

The cult of radionics catapulted into the national spotlight when Upton Sinclair became a believer. Sinclair, author of the classic novel exposé of the meatpacking industry *The Jungle*, was a household name when he lent his credibility to radionics by writing an article entitled "The House of Wonders" for *Pearson's Magazine* in June 1922. In the article, Sinclair praises and promotes Abrams and his methods:

> I decided to go to San Francisco and investigate. I planned to spend a day or two, but what I found there held me a couple of weeks, and it might have been months or even years, if urgent duties had not called me home. . . . This eager and excitable little Jewish doctor is either one of the greatest geniuses in the history of mankind, or else one of the greatest maniacs. But present him with a new idea, some way to verify or perfect his work, he pounces on it like a cat. He is a veritable incarnation of Nietzsche's phrase about the human soul, which "hungers for knowledge as the lion for his food." There is no experiment he will not try. . . . I speak the literal truth when I say that after a week in Abrams's clinic I had lost all feeling of the horror of the three dread diseases, tuberculosis, syphilis, and cancer.

Sinclair's piece led to a variety of articles in magazines across the country and in Britain. As radionics grew in popularity on both sides of the Atlantic, however, it also began to draw the critical eye of skeptics. Skeptics like the American Medical Association.

RADIONICS LOSES THE SIGNAL

In a brilliant plot, the AMA sent the blood of a healthy male guinea pig to a radionics practitioner for testing, concocting a backstory for the blood sample, claiming it was from a "Miss Bell." The test results came back saying that Miss Bell had cancer ("six ohms" worth of it), in addition to an infection of her left frontal sinus and a streptococcic infection of her left fallopian tube.

Scientific American followed suit, launching a yearlong investigation into radionics theories. The magazine published monthly updates between October 1923 and September 1924. The results:

> This committee finds that the claims advanced on behalf of the
> electronic reactions of Abrams, and of electronic practice in
> general, are not substantiated; and it is our belief that they have no
> basis in fact. In our opinion, the so-called electronic treatments are
> without value.

Damning words from a respected publication, followed shortly by a similar report in 1924 from a British committee who found the practice "scientifically unsound" and "ethically unjustified." The press also published a case of an elderly man who had visited the Mayo Clinic and was diagnosed with inoperable stomach cancer. The poor man turned to radionics and was told he was "completely cured" after the use of an Oscilloclast machine. He died a month later.

Sinclair, meanwhile, was quick to jump to Abrams's defense, writing:

> He has made the most revolutionary discovery of this or any other
> age. I venture to stake whatever reputation I ever hope to have that
> he has discovered the great secret of the diagnosis and cure of all
> major diseases.

Thankfully for Sinclair's future reputation, he also wrote a social justice masterpiece, so we can all just shuffle uncomfortably and turn a blind eye while he unleashes his fervent support for unabashed quackery. Despite Sinclair leaping to its defense, radionics lost much of its credibility from the *Scientific American* reports. Its founder, however, was no longer alive to witness the demise.

By the time Abrams died of pneumonia at age sixty, shortly after radionics became enormously successful, he was a very wealthy man. The Abrams estate was worth $2 million in 1924, a sad commentary on humanity's gullibility. In a curious postscript, Abrams claimed to be able to predict a person's death date with the Dynamizer. He correctly predicted that he would die in January 1924.

> ## PESTS BE GONE!
>
> T. Galen Hieronymus, an inventor in Kansas City, Missouri, built his own radionics device in 1949. The "Hieronymus machine" could allegedly detect "eloptic energy," which was said to emanate from all life. Hieronymus machines were used for agriculture, of all things, especially as alternatives to pesticides.
>
> For fun times, ask your local organic farmer if he used a Hieronymous machine!

THE FUTURE OF RADIONICS

In the vacuum created by Abrams's death, various other quack imitators quickly arose to fight for a share of the "healing via radio waves" market. None was more successful than Ruth B. Drown of Hollywood, California, who created her own radionics machines supposedly capable of healing anyone no matter where they were in the world.

Drown also found a willing audience for her quackery, treated some thirty-five thousand patients in her time, and sold her machines widely, particularly to other practitioners of fringe medicine. She also would take on cases without prompting.

In the early 1950s, film star Tyrone Power and his wife were injured in a car accident in Italy. Drown used one of her long-distance radio machines (the Model 300, for the curious) to send healing radio waves their way. Because her machines, like Abrams's Dynamizer, required some sort of sample from the patient, Drown used samples of the power couple's blood that she claimed to already have in her "library." (What? How? What?)

Tyrone and his wife recovered from the car accident and returned home to America. A bill for Drown's radionics services awaited them.

Radionics has always had a mystical element to it and, despite all the scientific evidence condemning the theory, it has managed to retain some devotees. Today, you can find radionics practitioners scattered around the United States. The focus, however, has shifted to the amplification of your thoughts into the greater consciousness of the universe. By using radionics, you can supposedly force your will on the world. You might use that ability to better your health or to find a lover or to get a great stock tip and make a pile of money. You can even make your own radionics machine. A simple Google search will bring up some free schematics. Maybe someday there will even be a Boy Scouts badge in "radionics."

Conventional medicine, meanwhile, obviously uses radio waves for communicating with dispatchers and paramedics. But many don't realize that radio frequency–driven heat energy is used to ablate or burn away problematic tissues. It can cure some types of heart arrhythmias, tumors, and varicose veins.

Perhaps somewhere, poor Upton Sinclair is feeling a little vindicated for his enthusiasm over the radio wave craze.

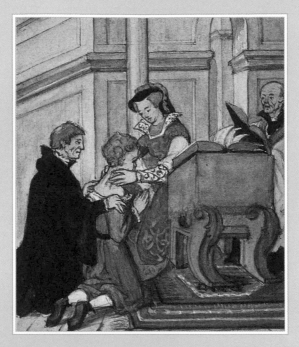

28

The King's Touch

Of Scrofula, *Macbeth*, Kingly Touching Ceremonies, a Miracle Horse, Medicinal Coins, and the Decayed Arm of Saint Louis

The medieval era was an ugly time to be alive. Without the benefit of modern medicine, all sorts of gruesome and disfiguring diseases rampaged their way through the European populace. Goiters, tumors, skin rashes, edema, cleft lips. But one of the worst of the skin diseases in Britain and France was scrofula, better known in its time as the "king's evil."

Scrofula (derived from the Latin word *scrofa*, meaning a breeding sow, because sows were thought to be susceptible to the disease) is a form of tuberculosis that infects the lymph nodes in your neck, producing large, unseemly growths that continue to expand with time. Rarely fatal, it is, however, quite disfiguring. Scrofula, as well as a host of other mysterious skin diseases, was typically referred to as the "king's evil" because it required the touch of a king to be cured.

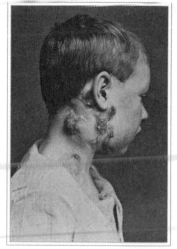

Scrofula in action.

So, you know, no worries. If you get a large, continually growing outbreak of scrofula on your neck, all you need to do is find a king. Once he's touched you, you're good to go. Good-bye disfiguring lumps.

Or so it seemed to the eleventh-century residents of Britain and France, when the practice of kings touching scrofula-infected peasantry became legitimized as a medical practice. As a demonstration of their divinely granted healing prowess, King Edward the Confessor of England (c. 1000–1066) and King Philip I of France (1052–1108) began holding public exhibitions of scrofula healing. Peasants burdened with the disease gathered at a pompous royal ceremony where the kings touched the victims, theoretically curing them.

Parliament member Samuel Pepys described such a ceremony in 1660, a few hundred years later, when Charles II sat on the throne:

> His Majesty began first to touch for ye evil according to custom,
> thus: his Majesty sitting under his state in the Banqueting-House,
> the surgeon cause the sick to be brought or led up to the throne,
> where they, kneeling, ye king strokes their faces or cheeks
> with both his hands at once, at which instant, a chaplain in his
> formalities, says, "He put his hands upon them and healed them."

It didn't hurt that, if left untreated, some cases of scrofula will seem to head into remission. Or at least with enough frequency to make it seem like the king's touch could have been a major contributor to—or the sole reason for—a cure.

Another reason for the popularity of king's touch ceremonies among the British peasantry was the chance to receive a special gold coin dubbed an "Angel" for the image of St. Michael minted on its front. After being touched by the king, the peasant was given this special coin, first minted

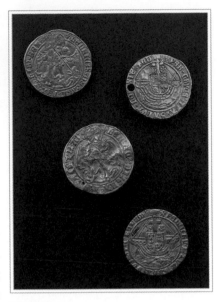

Magic coins.

in 1465. These souvenirs would go on to become prized family heirlooms and were assumed to maintain a little bit of that kingly healing magic inside them. People would wear them on special chains around their necks and rub the coins over their bodies when they were suffering from ailments.

It's not difficult to imagine that physical contact with a king—or queen, for that matter—combined with the receipt of a "magic coin," might have inspired awe and wonder in the medieval peasantry. Deeply entrenched in a serfdom economy and without the benefit of modern education, such an experience could quite conceivably generate a powerful placebo effect, possibly helping scrofula symptoms to retreat.

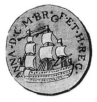

More magic coins.

The kings and queens, meanwhile, do not appear to have been concerned about catching scrofula themselves. Granted it's pretty easy to just, you know, touch yourself if you're a king and cure the disease before the rest of the population realizes you have it. But can you imagine the public relations nightmare if a king who practiced the touch came down with scrofula himself? Because the practice died down before we understood how contagious diseases spread, it's safe to assume that the kings and queens who participated in the ceremony genuinely believed that there wasn't a chance in hell they could catch scrofula from their subjects. It was really just a happy fluke of history (from the monarchy's perspective, anyway) that none of them, apparently, ever did.

KINGLY LEGITIMACY VIA TOUCHING, OR TOO LEGIT TO QUIT

The royal touch even makes an appearance in Shakespeare's *Macbeth*, when a doctor informs Malcolm and Macduff that King Edward the Confessor is busy touching scrofula patients at the moment:

> **Malcolm:** Comes the king forth, I pray you?
> **The Doctor:** Ay, sir, there are a crew of wretched souls,
> That stay his cure. Their malady convinces
> The great assay of art, but at his touch—
> Such sanctity hath heaven given his hand—
> They presently amend.

In fact, the royal touch is one of the reasons Malcolm and Macduff enlist King Edward the Confessor—a "true king" because of his divinely granted healing powers—to help them overthrow Macbeth. Shakespeare was definitely ripping from the headlines here: Throughout history, the king's touch had the extraordinary political benefit of legitimizing a king's rule in the eyes of the public.

After Edward the Confessor and Philip I in the eleventh century, the ability to cure scrofula by the laying on of hands became viewed as divinely inherited. Only the "true king" could do it. Predictably, the ability appeared to pass down through the strict familial descent of parent to child, thus helping to preserve dynastic control over a kingdom.

The divine right to rule, demonstrated in part by the healing powers of the king's touch, became such an important aspect of kingly legitimacy that English rulers kept it up for seven hundred years and French rulers for eight hundred years. One might argue that you can track the popularity of a monarchy by how desperately it clings to its royal legitimacy. It's almost as if the populace gets reminded of the royal touch whenever the king needs a boost in his approval rating. Funny that.

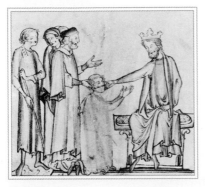

Touched by a King.

Take England. With the notable exception of Henry IV—who touched a staggering fifteen hundred victims in a single ceremony—rulers practiced the king's touch somewhat indifferently, stroking only a handful of patients each year, until a major spike in the seventeenth century. Then things got serious. Charles II (1630–1685) opened the floodgates, touching some ninety-two thousand scrofula patients during his twenty-five year reign, averaging about thirty-seven hundred people per year.

And why might he have wanted to touch so many people? Well, the monarchy was on pretty shaky grounds in those days. Charles's own father, Charles I, was beheaded in 1649, during the English Civil War. Charles II was subsequently defeated in battle by Oliver Cromwell in 1651, fleeing to safety across the Channel to mainland Europe. England then spent nine years toying with the English Commonwealth, before finally inviting Charles II back from exile in 1660 in the turmoil following Cromwell's death.

So the king had a clear and obvious legitimacy objective, and he could hardly get scrofula patients through the palace gates fast enough. As in the wise words of the late-twentieth-century bard, MC Hammer, Charles II was indeed too legit to quit.

And yet, all the scrofula-stroking in the world couldn't prevent the fall of Charles's House of Stuart when Queen Anne died in 1714. But the scrappy family wouldn't let exile and the Hanoverian monarchy keep them down. They persistently clung to their claims on the British throne, launching several Jacobite rebellions in the eighteenth century. Their followers also spread the rumor that the Stuarts could still perform the miracle of the king's touch. ("See, *our* king can still cure scrofula with his touch. Isn't it obvious that God favors him and he has the divine right to sit on the British throne?") It didn't help: All of the Jacobite rebellions, although romantically entangled with simmering conceptions of Scottish nationalism, ended in failure.

France, meanwhile, practiced a kind of king's-touch-on-steroids. From the late Middle Ages onward, the ritual was incorporated into the coronation ceremonies of French kings, a nice way to cement divine right from the get-go.

The king's touch reached its zenith of popularity in seventeenth-century France—when Louis XIV celebrated Easter in 1680 not with an Easter egg hunt at Versailles (party!), but by touching sixteen hundred scrofulous patients. Even as the practice declined in the eighteenth century, Louis XV certainly did his part to keep the flame alive, bringing the number-of-scrofula-patients-touched-by-the-king-in-one-sitting record to the staggering figure of twenty-four hundred people.

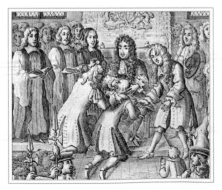

It's a little different, isn't it, than Queen Elizabeth II waving at the crowd from her motorcade?

Engraving of the King's Touch.

CAN'T GET THE REAL THING?
TRY THESE KING'S TOUCH KNOCKOFFS!

———

A very real problem faced by peasants afflicted with the king's evil: If you have a disease that only a king can cure, you're kind of dependent on meeting him. Unless you were able to travel to London or Paris for a king's touch ceremony—in the days before EasyJet and Ryanair—you were flat out of luck. If you were naturally lucky, scrofula symptoms might abate on their own. Or, you could also find alternative healers to kings. Alternative healers such as horses.

Alexander Shields, a Scottish nonconformist, wrote in his diary in 1688 of a special horse in the Annandale region of Scotland who could cure scrofula by licking the sores of the victims: "I was told, by an eye witness, of a horse in or about the foot of Annandale that cures the King's evil by licking the sore, unto which many country people resort from all quarters."

What a boon that licking horse must have been for the poor people of remote Scotland who had almost zero chance of ever meeting the king in person. And what a boon that licking horse must have been to the farmer who owned her. That farmer must have been a canny businessman with the spirit of a quack doctor, generating a tidy profit by granting access to his miracle horse. (How the horse was convinced to lick the growths in the first place has been lost to history.)

Also a bit remote for a royal touch pilgrimage, Ireland had its own alternative in the mid-seventeenth century. In 1662, an Irish faith healer with the incredible name of Valentine Greatrakes (aka "the Stroker," seriously) came to fame, claiming the ability to heal scrofula by touching afflicted patients. This, despite the very obvious fact that Valentine was not a king. Owing to the difficulty of Irish peasantry traveling to London to be touched by the actual king (and undoubtedly helped by the traditional Irish republican view on the monarchy in general), Greatrakes, well, raked it in. Greatly. For three years, masses of people assembled wherever he appeared for the opportunity to be touched by him. Greatrakes eventually drew the ire of the Bishop's Court at Lismore, who banned him from performing medical cures for the age-old reason of "not having a proper license."

That didn't stop him. In 1666, Greatrakes hopped across the pond to England and continued to touch scrofula patients as he toured across the country. Eventually, Charles II heard of Greatrakes and summoned him to appear in Whitehall to demonstrate his abilities. Despite

OTHER KINGLY GIFTS

Although the French and English rulers were unique among European monarchy in their ability to cure scrofula, they were not the only aristocrats thought to contain innate healing powers. The Hapsburgs of Austria could allegedly cure stuttering by kissing you on the mouth. And the monarchs of Castile in Spain could exorcise demons by praying to God and making the sign of the cross near you.

So, if you were a demon-possessed stutterer with a bad case of scrofula, you could cure all of your ailments by simply embarking on a Grand Tour of Europe.

And that might be the best remedy we've ever heard suggested.

a lingering doubt over the efficacy of the Stroker's stroking (and despite a deep personal enthusiasm for his own royal touching abilities), Charles II surprisingly did not forbid Greatrakes from advertising his services, and he let the Irish faith healer continue to travel around England unmolested. The king had more important things to worry about such as the ongoing Second Anglo-Dutch War.

After igniting quite a lot of controversy in the British press about his touching abilities (Robert Boyle, founder of modern chemistry, even came out as a Greatrakes supporter), the Stroker returned to Ireland in 1667, where he took up farming.

But if you couldn't find an Irish faith healer, or a living king, perhaps we could interest you in . . . a dead one? The French were so enamored by the practice that a belief sprang up that the touch of a king could even cure scrofula *from beyond the grave*. (Pause here for the sound of thunder to subside.)

The decayed arm of Louis IX (1214–1270), who had the extra sparkle of being a dead saint in addition to a dead king, was believed to retain the healing power of the king's touch. Inspired pilgrims from across Europe trekked to a monastery in Spain where the king was buried with one abiding hope: to have their scrofula touched by the skeletal arm of a long dead king.

Losing Touch

When William and Mary took the English throne in 1689, the king's touch fell out of favor entirely. With the continued growth of a Protestantism in England that was strongly anti-Catholic and strongly anti-superstition, the new rulers refused to grant requests for the royal touch. The practice was beginning to be associated, negatively, with Catholicism. William even went so far as to throw down a seventeenth-century burn on a petitioner suffering from scrofula who asked for William's touch. His response? "God grant you better health . . . and better sense."

Ouch. Just what some poor bastard suffering from scrofula wants to hear from his king.

Queen Anne briefly reintroduced the practice during her short reign. In March 1712, Anne performed the ritual for the last time and, in a historical footnote under the "strange coincidence" heading, the last scrofula patient to receive Anne's touch was none other than a little toddler named Samuel Johnson. Yes, *that* Samuel Johnson, the one who would later become famous for writing the first modern dictionary of the English language. Alas, with the passing of

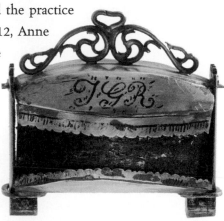

A lodestone that Queen Anne used during ceremonies when she didn't want to touch peasants directly.

the Stuarts (and their efforts to legitimize their claims to the throne), so too did the practice of the king's touch pass from England.

Meanwhile, in France, the practice also started to decline in the eighteenth century. The French population, awash in the glow of the Age of Enlightenment, began to doubt the efficacy of the king's touch. The

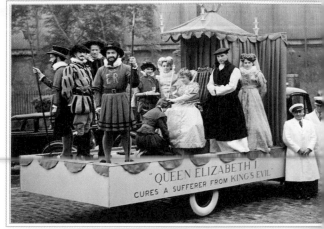

A royal reenactment: The queen dishes out cures from the back of a lorry.

scientific revolution had catapulted reason to the top of the list of "ways to evaluate the world around you," and in France the *Siècle des Lumières* led to a fast-growing opposition to an absolute monarchy. An example of the rising skepticism of kingly powers was captured by Voltaire, ever the witty observer, who noted that a mistress of Louis XIV died from scrofula despite "being very well touched by the king."

The occasional monarch would continue to resurrect the tradition until 1825, when Charles X touched 121 scrofula patients at his coronation, the last time a French monarch publicly employed the practice. Although, to be fair, the French monarchy was just about over.

Although France no longer has a monarchy, we can always hold out hope for England. Perhaps once Prince William assumes the kingly mantle, he will decide to reintroduce the practice for the twenty-first century. Legions of fans would willingly infect themselves with scrofula just for that very opportunity.

The Eye Care Hall of Shame

Perfect vision is a rare miracle; much of the world's population struggles with conditions such as nearsightedness, far-sightedness, astigmatism, or presbyopia. Despite the recent trend of vanity glasses and frames-as-fashion-statements, for many of us who suffer from imperfect vision, we'd love to be able to wake up in the morning and not have to reach for our glasses before we can see the alarm clock beside the bed.

Many a keen businessman has been aware of that very desire, leading to a variety of quack products and theories promising easy (and sometimes humorous) fixes for complex vision problems. Like most examples of quackery, the only person who tended to benefit from these products and theories was the manufacturer or salesman himself.

THE BATES SYSTEM OF EYE EXERCISES

Against all evidence to the contrary, New York ophthalmologist William Horatio Bates thought that wearing eyeglasses was a bad idea for people with vision problems. To improve your eyesight, you simply had to perform a series of eye exercises, such as swinging your eyes from object to object, palming your eyeballs, and visualizing "pure black." The Bates Method was an enormous hit in the 1920s and '30s, spawning numerous quacks in its wake and attracting a slavish devotion, for no obvious reason, in Nazi Germany. Happily, the Bates Method was never adopted by the DMV.

NOSE WRITING WITH ALDOUS HUXLEY

One of the most enthusiastic adopters of the Bates Method was Aldous Huxley, English author of *Brave New World*, who had been haunted by vision problems all of his life. Huxley even wrote a book about his conversion, *The Art of Seeing*, which was reluctantly published by Harper in 1942 and remains the problem child in Huxley's literary canon. Among other absurdities, Huxley recommends the practice of "nose writing," that is, imagining your nose is a pencil and then writing an imaginary signature in the air with your nose pencil . . . as a way to improve your eyesight.

GAYELORD HAUSER'S WONDER FOODS

Gayelord Hauser, tireless self-promoter and creator of one of the first celebrity diets, was one of the better-known quacks to follow in Bates's footsteps. Hauser's book *Keener Vision without Glasses* basically co-opted the Bates method as a way to promote and sell Hauser's dietary products. You could improve your eyesight if you performed eye exercises . . . and consistently ate the "wonder foods" that were conveniently sold by Hauser's own company. (Note: Gayelord Hauser–approved "wonder foods" included yogurt, brewer's yeast, powdered skim milk, wheat germ, and blackstrap molasses.)

GALVANIC SPECTACLES

A steampunk's dream come true, the "galvanic spectacles" from circa 1905 had dark green lenses and a plastic frame concealing a secondary, metal frame underneath with electric wiring. The glasses purported to send a "continuous stream of electricity to the optic nerve," the benefits of which, the manufacturers assumed, would be obvious to the consumer. What was less obvious to the manufacturers was the fact that the optic nerve isn't actually in the eyeball; it's behind the eyeball, deep in the skull. (Note: Electric shocks to your eyes may give you a lot of steampunk cred, but they will not improve your vision.)

DR. ISAAC THOMPSON'S CELEBRATED EYE WATER

First patented and marketed by Dr. Isaac Thompson (not actually a doctor) in Connecticut in 1795, this general cure-all for eye complaints was still being sold in the twentieth century. No one really knew its ingredients, however, until the passage of the Pure Food and Drug Act in 1906.

The real reason for its long-standing popularity?

Opium.

JUST LOOK IN THE MIRROR

A bizarre notion that the irises of the eyes could be used to diagnose patients sprang up in the nineteenth century when Hungarian physician Ignaz von Peczely observed a similar iris pattern in the eyes of both a man with a broken leg

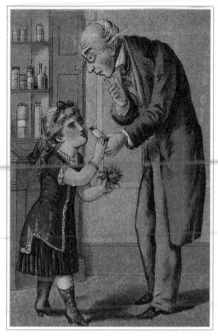

Nothing to see here, just a leering old man presenting strange medicinal eye water to an innocent young girl.

. . . and an *owl* with a broken leg. Why Peczely didn't chock this up to chance, why Peczely had an owl in the first place, and why he was gazing so intensely into the eyes of both man and bird that he was able to make this kind of comparative analysis, remain lost to history.

Regardless, the practice of iridology (still going strong) sprang up in the wake of Peczely's . . . discovery.

The Cancer Cure Hall of Shame

Cancer is an illness that seemingly changes the unchangeable constant of our very self—our DNA. It begins when one of our own cells transforms irrevocably into something that stops acting, well, normally human. It multiplies, unstoppable in its quest to double and double again, to the point of killing us. Cancer isn't contagious; it doesn't seek to find other hosts and spread to others, like viruses or bacteria. It is simply a one-job hit-man.

Hippocrates coined the terms *carcinos* and *carcinoma* to describe malignant tumors in the fourth century BCE. Both terms refer to the word for *crab* because many tumors have creeping projections that resemble crab legs emanating from the center. Sometimes the surface of the tumor resembles a crab carapace; sometimes the lancinating pain feels like a crab's pincers. By the time Celsus showed up in the first century BCE, the word had been officially translated into its current iteration.

Cancer has been fought in a lot of unfortunate ways. Because we don't have all the cures yet, quacks continue to abound in their efforts to prey on the desperate—just take a gander at some of the worst treatments you'd never want to try.

ANIMALS

In the long line of "like cures like" treatments, this one takes the crab cake, so to speak. In the second century CE, Galen suggested burning crabs and smearing ashes and crab bits onto tumors with a feather. But crabs weren't the only victims. In the Middle Ages, one method recommended holding a freshly killed rabbit, puppy, kitten, or lamb against the tumor. The idea was that the cancer was akin to a ravenous wolf and would feed off the sacrificed animal rather than the human. Poor critters! In the eighteenth century, such treatments included fox lungs, lizard's blood, and crocodile dung, along with the usual but useless modalities, like leeching.

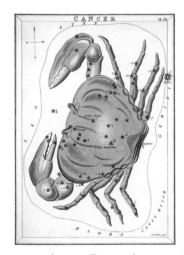

Cancer—a crab, a constellation, a plague on society.

GRAPES

In 1925, Johanna Brandt introduced her Grape Cure. It's a pretty simple idea—you fast for a few days, and then use enemas, and then eat seven meals of grapes every day for two weeks. Grape juice enemas, douches, poultices, and gargles were recommended, too. As if once weren't enough, the American Cancer Society debunked the juicy practice four separate times (the last in 2000).

SHARK CARTILAGE

You might have heard that sharks can't get cancer. In 1992, William Lane and Linda Comac published a book called exactly that—*Sharks Don't Get Cancer*—and a roar of interest came with it. Anyone who read the book could pretty much say, "Why yes, I don't know any sharks with cancer! Not a one!" Perhaps if patients were treated with shark cartilage and whatever magic mysteries it possessed cured cancer, then oncologists across the world would be out of a job. Want to know the results of several scientific studies? (Hint: Oncologists still have a job.)

In any case, it really did seem an interesting idea, until biologists pointed out this sad fact: Sharks *do* get cancer.

Mic drop.

ZAPPERS

Royal Raymond Rife was an inventor who claimed his beam ray, the Rife Frequency Generator, could kill the microbes he thought caused human illness, including cancer. He believed he could target these microbes, which—unbeknownst to microbiologists—apparently vibrated and shot off colorful auras (sounding about as believable as rainbow unicorns). The machine was a large black box with dials and a glass "ray tube" that looked like a lightbulb sticking out the side. Though all this occurred in the 1930s, modern Rife devices are still on the market today for thousands of dollars, and several sellers have been convicted of felony health fraud.

CYANIDE

In the 1970s, a treatment called laetrile was the hot new commodity. Occasionally called vitamin B-17 (it's not a vitamin), laetrile is a semisynthetic form of amygdalin, a cyanide-containing compound found in apricot pits and other seeds. Laetrile supporters claimed that it could somehow directly target and kill cancer cells, leaving the healthy ones alone. The claim was false, and subjects taking it in a formal clinical trial ended up with cyanide toxicity. So much for the idea that cancer might be a deficiency in vitamin B-17. Thanks, but no, humans aren't lacking in cyanide, and we don't really want more. Really.

Laetrile has fallen out of favor in the last two decades, but for those diehard vitamin B-17 lovers, it's still available on the Internet and at a few shady across-the-border clinics.

WHAT ACTUALLY WORKS

Philadelphia physician Benjamin Rush once remarked, "I am disposed to believe that there does not exist in the vegetable kingdom an antidote to cancers." He might have been surprised to find that yew trees and periwinkle plants would become sources of two powerhouse chemotherapeutics—paclitaxel and vinca alkaloids—that

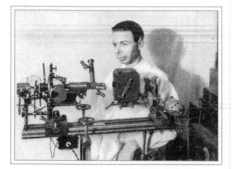

Royal Rife in 1931 with an early microscope invention.

treat a variety of cancers. Many would be shocked to find that arsenic, commonly found in dangerous and useless old nostrums, is now an important treatment for one type of leukemia.

Today, we battle malignancies with chemotherapy that includes targeted biologic therapies. There's hormone blockade for hormonally driven cancers, monoclonal antibodies that target cancer cells, and, most recently, directed immunotherapy that activates our own immune system to kill cancer cells. Surgery is now far more precise and safe thanks to antisepsis and a modern understanding of anatomy. And though radiation can cause cancer, contemporary radiation oncologists have a keen understanding of the physics of radiation, and they wield improved technology to target treatment areas with precise doses. Make no mistake, we have a lot more work to do, but we no longer live in those helpless eras where you just ate grapes and hoped for the best.

Acknowledgments

One sunny morning at a cafe in San Diego, April Genevieve Tucholke turned to us and said, "You should write a book together." A very special thanks to April for launching us on this hugely enjoyable ride.

To Eric Myers, our agent for this book, who saw the diamond-in-the-rough of our proposal, thanks for making this possible.

To Sam O'Brien, our editor, and the rest of the brilliant team at Workman— thank you for finding a home for *Quackery*, and making it polish up to a high shine. This was seriously fun. Seriously weird sometimes, but seriously fun.

A very special thanks to the librarians and staff at the University of Nebraska Medical Center McGoogan Library of Medicine. John Schleicher provided a wonderful tour through the historical archives. Mary Helms paved the way there and has been so supportive of this project. Cameron Boettcher shared some amazing photos with us. And to all the librarians who searched out the article requests for things that included "cannibalism" and "arsenic poisoning"—thank you for not calling the Police Department.

Lydia Kang

To my best friend and partner in life, Bernie Su, who worked as my unpaid editor and consultant. To my children—thanks for never freaking out when I yelped out random, bizarre things during the writing of this manuscript. To Dr. Chang-Wuk Kang, and my brother, Dr. Richard Kang, you both embody grace, the intelligence, and strength in your work and lives. To my mom, Kyong-Ja, who never stops looking out for me—love from me to you. Alice, for the never-ending sisterly support. To Dana, Ohsang—huge hugs, always. And to my gaggle of nieces and nephews—your auntie is weird and you don't care and I love ya for that. To all my Su family—your love, support, and curiosity are always appreciated.

I have so many friends in the medical world who offered advice and support—Angela Hawkins, Chris Bruno, Gale Etherton, and Fedja Rochling, amongst many others. My clinic support staff and my colleagues—thank you for taking such great care of my wonderful patients with me. Lois Colburn, thank you for your gift of quacky books and your enthusiasm. To Cynthia Leitich Smith, for your time and expertise. Sydnee Schmidt, for all the bibliography help, and Emalee Napier, for keeping the world around me organized. Lots of love to Dushana, Tonya, Maurene, Cindy, Anna, Ellen, Ariane, and many others who supported me during this busy year. To Sarah Fine, who is my writing rock. Rock on, darling.

And finally to Nate, my partner in poisonous crime—you are the chillest dude I know, and you're beyond awesome. Let's get dinner with our SO's soon, okay?

NATE PEDERSEN

Lydia Kang—thanks for your mind-blowing efficiency, speed, and medical accuracy. You were the perfect coauthor. Let's do this again sometime.

Paul Collins and Scott Carney for generously offering advice when I first started freelancing as a journalist. And Simon Winchester for telling me to stop freelancing and try writing a book instead.

James Danky for all the support through the years.

Rebecca Rego-Barry of *Fine Books & Collections* magazine, for the writerly support, editorial input, and for providing a home for so many of my articles.

Deschutes Public Library.

Deschutes County Historical Society & Museum.

Kelly Cannon-Miller for co-conspiring.

Thomas Pedersen for always being there and always cheering me on.

April Genevieve Tucholke for too many damn things to name.

In Memory of
Einar and Beulah Pedersen, Neil Whitehead, Norman Kane,
and especially my mother, Donna Pedersen.

A

abdominal pain, 193
Abrams, Albert, 304–12
abstinence, 246
acrodynia, 4, 14
addiction treatments, 36,
    101. *see also* alcoholism
aging, 239
Aiken's Tonic Pills, 28
al-Birumi, 124
alchemists, 8, 37, 39, 40, 42,
    284
alcohol, 66–67, 80, 96, 102–4,
    105–14
alcoholism, 23–24, 36,
    40–42, 204–5
Aldini, Giovanni, 272–73
Aldobrandino of Siena, 113
Alexander III, Pope, 133
All Products Unlimited, 79
Allan's Anti-Fat, 268
allergies, 19
Allsopp's Ales, 80
Alvarez, Walter C., 172
ambergris, 237
American Chemical
    Society, 49–50
American Vegetarian Party,
    263
amphetamines, 268
amputations, 185, 186–89
amygdalin, 327–28
anal leeches, 214, 216
Andromachus, 126
anemia, 79
anesthesia/anesthetics, 84,
    100, 106, 194, 195–208,
    290
animal magnetism, 281–91
animal-derived medicines,
    233–43
animals
    cancer and, 326, 327
    cannibalism, 221–32

corpse medicine, 221–32
    fasting, 255–68
    leeches, 211–20
    sex, 244–54
anise, 57
Anne, Queen, 136, 319, 322
Antabuse, 24
anthropophagy, 221–32
anticoagulants, 220
antidiarrheals, 84, 119
antidotes, 116, 120, 124–26
anti-inflammatories, 234
antimalarials, 28
antimony, 15–24, 161
antipsychotics, 150
antisepsis/antiseptics, 106,
    190, 328
apomorphine, 22
apoplectic attacks, 229
Appelgate, Ada, 27
appendicitis, 164
Arabian mummies, 231
argyria, 42
arrow wounds, 185
arsenic, 21, 25–34, 328
Art of Seeing, The (Huxley),
    324
arthritis, 47
artificial respiration, 90
Asclepius, Rod of, 14
asphyxiation, 196
aspirin, 70
asthma, 19, 70, 94
atropine, 126
auric fever, 38
autointoxication, 165–66,
    167, 169, 170, 171, 172,
    193
aversion therapy, 22, 23–24
Avicenna, 62, 64–65

B

Bacon, Roger, 107–8
bad air, 166

Bailey, William, 49–50, 53
Bailey Radium Laboratory,
    45
baldness, 208, 275
Balzac, Honoré de, 189
barbers, 133–34
Bates, William Horatio, 324
Bates Method, 324
Batmanghelidj, Fereydoon,
    181
Bayer Laboratories, 70, 71
beard generators, 208
beaver testicles, 237
Bee Brand White Pine and
    Tar Cough Syrup, 199
beer, 22, 80, 113–14
Beerbohm, Max, 27
Bell, Benjamin, 188
Bennett, John Hughes,
    138–39, 220
Bennett, Kate Brewington,
    32–33
Benzedrine, 268
benzodiazepines, 205
Berthold, Andreas, 116–17,
    119–22
beta-phenylisopropylamine,
    268
bezoars, 124–25
biases, ix
bile, 5, 9, 17, 131, 167
bismarsen, 33
Black Death. *see* plague
bladder stones, 191, 202
blister beetle (*Lytta
    vesicatoria*), 159–60
blistering, 23, 151–62
blood, coughing up, 231
blood clotting, prevention
    of, 243
blood drinking, 223–25
blood transfusions, 232
bloodletting, 7, 129–39,
    212–13

Bloomer, Amelia, 177
bloomers, 177
blue light, 292–95
blue mass, 9
blue skin, 42
blue vitriol (copper sulfate),
    22
body dysmorphic disorder,
    194
Boerhaave, Herman, 40
boils, 222
bone marrow, 226, 230
Bosch, Hieronymus, 143
bottled water, 182
Bowen device, 207
Boyle, Robert, 321
Braid, James, 290–91
brain fog, 301
brain inflammation, 212
brains, 228–29
Brandt, Johanna, 326
brandy, 109, 111–13
Breatharianism, 264
Brinkley, John Romulus,
    238, 241–42
Brodie, Ben, 92
broken bones, 185, 227
bronchitis, 79
Brooklyn Enigma, 258, 259
Brooks, Wiley, 264
Broussais, François-Joseph-
    Victor, 218
Brown, Isaac Baker, 57
Browne, Edward, 224
Brown-Séquard, Charles-
    Édouard, 159
bruising, 231
Brunschwig, Hieronymus,
    156
bubonic plague. see plague
Bulgakov, Mikhail, 241
bullet wounds, 156–58, 192
Burckhardt, Gottlieb,
    144–45

burns, 237
Burroughs, Stanley, 262
Burroughs, William S., 254
Byers, Eben, 44–45, 52–53
Byron, Lord, 136

C

caduceus, 14
caffeine, 82
calicos vomitorii, 20
calomel, 4–7, 12, 13–14
Camel advertisements, 94
camphor, 162
cancer
    arsenic and, 28, 34
    enemas and, 170, 172
    fasting and, 265
    gold and, 43
    hall of shame for, 326–28
    mumia and, 231
    radium and, 46–47, 51, 54
    tobacco and, 85, 94
cannibalism, 221–32
Canon of Medicine
    (Avicenna), 64
cantharidin, 160
capsaicin, 162
carbon dioxide, 196–97
carbon monoxide, 199
carbonic acid gas, 196
cardiac arrhythmias, 208
Carman, A. R., 158, 159
carmine, 243
carotid artery, 192–93
castoreum, 237
Catherine de' Medici, 87
Cato, 106
cattle distemper virus, 16
cautery, 151–62, 185, 187
Celestial Bed, 280
Celsus, 22, 156, 157, 326
Ceruleo, 300
charcoal, activated, 24, 126
Charles I, 318

Charles II, 136, 229, 315,
    318–19, 321
Charles V, 156
Charles X, 323
chelation therapies, 24
chemotherapeutics, 328
Chevallier, Dr., 31
chewing, excessive, 268
childbed fever, 190
childbirth. see also
    pregnancy
    animal remedies for,
        57–58
    bloodletting and, 135
    brandy and, 112
    human skin and, 227
children
    cocaine and, 101
    gin and, 109
    leeches and, 219
    lobotomies and, 150
    opiates and, 62–63
    strychnine and, 4
    tobacco smoke and, 91
    tonsillectomies and, 194
Chinese water torture, 180
chloroform, 197–99, 202
chlorpromazine, 150
cholera, 68, 91, 166, 170, 300
Christian IV, 228
Christian Science, 287
chrysiasis, 43
circumcision, 194
Clark, William, 12
Clark Stanley's Snake Oil
    Liniment, 234, 236
Claudius, 17
clay, 115–23
Cleopatra, 126
clitoridectomies, 57
clysters, 163–72
Cobain, Kurt, 254
Cobbett, William, 7, 138
Coca Beef Tonic, 102

coca leaves, 98–99, 104
coca wine, 96, 102–4
Coca-Cola, 96, 104
cocaine, 95–104
Cocoanuts, The, 241
coffee enema, 171, 172
Cogan, Thomas, 90
coins, 316
cold shower, 178
cold water cure, 173–83
cold water pour, 179
colds, 237
colectomies, 193
colic, 204
colloidal gold, 42, 43
color therapy, 298–301
Columbus, Battle of, 95–96
Comac, Linda, 327
Compound Sulphur Lozenges, 28
Confessions of an English Opium-Eater (De Quincey), 67
constipation, 4, 5, 12, 81, 106, 164, 166–67, 170, 171, 193, 250–51, 275, 296
continuous hot bath, 179
convulsions, 284
Cook, James, 20
Cooper, Astley, 142, 191
Cooper, Bransby, 191
copper sulfate (blue vitriol), 22
corpse medicine, 221–32, 321–22
cosmetics, 21, 32–33, 49
counter-irritation, 23, 158–59, 162
crabs, 326
Cramp, Arthur J., 172
Crampton, Philip, 217
Creamy Snuff, 92

Creighton, Mary Frances, 25–26, 27, 30
Crohn's disease, 178
Cromwell, Oliver, 318
Cruden, Alexander, 135
Culpeper, Nicholas, 38
cupping, 137, 139
Curie, Marie and Pierre, 46
Cutting the Stone (Bosch), 143
cyanide, 327–28

D
Daffy's Elixir, 62
Darwin, Charles, 29, 178
Davy, Humphry, 199–200
De Quincey, Thomas, 67
deafness, 291
defibrillator, 279
dehydration, 181
demons, 321
depression, 164, 193, 302
detoxing, 262
Devi, Kunjarani, 82
Dewey, Edward, 260–61
Dexedrine, 268
diabetes, 47, 94, 243, 296
diacetylmorphine, 69–70
diarrhea, 64, 68, 199, 204
Dieffenbach, Johann Friedrich, 192
diethyl ether, 202
dinitrophenol, 268
Dinshah Health Society, 302
Dioscorides, 108, 118, 195
diphtheria, 161
directed immunotherapy, 328
dirt eating (geophagy), 117, 121
disinfectants, tobacco smoke as, 91
distillation, 111

Dormer, Anne, 229
douche, 180
Dover, Thomas, 67
Dover's Powder, 67
Doyle, Arthur Conan, 103
Dr. Isaac Thompson's Celebrated Eye Water, 325
Dr. Jekyll and Mr. Hyde (Stevenson), 102
Dr. Kelly's Remedy, 204–5
Dr. Koester's Antigas Tablets, 81
Dr. Moffett's Teethina Powder, 4
Dr. Newman's Obesity Pills, 266
Dr. Rush's Bilious Pills/ Thunderbolts, 12
Dr. Scott's Electric Hair Brush, 275–76
Dr. Young's Ideal Rectal Dilators, 250–51
drenching, 180
Dreser, Heinrich, 70
dripping machine, 180
drooling, 5–6
dropped kidneys, 193
dropsy, 164, 167
Drown, Ruth B., 312–13
drowning, 88–90, 164
dry eyes, 243
Dully, Howard, 150
Dumas, Alexandre, 103
dyes, arsenic in, 33
Dynamizer, 306–8, 310, 312
dysentery, 68, 69, 120, 169, 170, 300
dyspepsia, 258, 277
Dyspepsia Bitters, 79

E
earth, 115–26
Easton's Syrup, 80–81

Ebers Papyrus, 56, 62

Eddy, Mary Baker, 287

Edison, Thomas, 103, 296

Edward, King, 298

Edward the Confessor, 315, 317

egg donation, 232

Einstein, Albert, 253–54

electric baths, 278–79

electric belts, 275, 276–77

electrical brushes, 275–76

electrical corsets, 273, 276

electricity, 271–80

Electro Thermal Company, 207

electrocardiogram (EKG), 279

electrocautery, 162

electromechanical vibrator, 248

electronic muscle stimulator (EMS) machines, 208

electrophysiology, 200

elements

    antimony, 15–24

    arsenic, 25–34

    gold, 35–43

    mercury, 3–14

    radium, 44–58

    radon, 44–58

elephantiasis, 225

elixir vitae, 223

eloptic energy, 312

emanators, 48

emesis (vomiting), 16–18

emetics, 17, 22, 126. *see also* antimony

emphysema, 94

encephalitis, 161

enema bulb, 163

enemas, 77, 88–90, 163–72, 178, 326

epidurals, 205

epiglottitis, 136

epilepsy, 38, 143, 185, 212, 214, 223, 224, 226, 228–29, 231, 237, 291

Erasistratus, 131, 138

erectile dysfunction, 275, 277

erethism, mercurial, 6, 9, 13

escharotics, 28

Esdaile, James, 289–90

ethanol, 126, 145

ether inhalation, 198, 202–5

ethyl ether, 202

everlasting pills, 20–21

evidence-based medicine, 219–20

evil spirits, 213

Executive Fitness Products, 208

exorcism, 321

eyes, 120, 324–25

F

Fancher, Mollie, 258, 259

fasting, 255–68

Fasting Cure, The (Sinclair), 265

Fasting for the Cure of Disease (Hazzard), 255

Father Hell (Hell, Maximilian), 283, 284

fatuity, 135

Fellows, James, 79

Fellows & Company, 79–80

Fellows' Compound Syrup of Hypophosphites, 79–80

fentanyl, 205

Ferrand, Jacques, 134, 159

fevers, 16, 120, 161, 212, 225, 274

Ficino, Marsilio, 223–24

filariasis, 289

Finsen, Niels Ryberg, 296

Fioravanti, Leonardo, 224

flatulence, 212

Flaubert, Gustave, 277

fleam, 132

Fletcher, Horace, 268

Fludd, Robert, 222

Food and Drug Administration (FDA), ix

Forster, George, 271–73

Fouquier, Pierre, 76–77

Fowler, Thomas, 28

Fowler's Solution, 28–30, 32, 34

Fracastoro, Girolamo, 12

Franklin, Benjamin, 273, 289

Freeman, Walter, 141, 146, 148–50

Freud, Sigmund, 100

fruit fly, 236

fulminate of gold, 39–40

Fundamentals of Nature Cure, The (Shelton), 261, 263

G

Gage, Phineas, 147

Galen, 5, 10, 64, 107, 119, 131, 134–35, 165, 168, 213, 246, 326

gallbladders, 226

Galvani, Luigi, 273

galvanic spectacles, 324–25

galvanism, 271–74, 277

gamma rays, 49

gangrene, 161, 186, 188

Garfield, James, 192

garlic, 22, 57

Geber, 37

Geiger counter, 53

gelatin, 243

genever, 110

geophagy, 117, 121

George II, 21

germ theory, 190
Gerson, Max, 170–71
Ghadiali, Dinshah P., 298–302
Gibson's Linseed Licorice, 199
Gilbert, William, 273
gin, 108–11
gin blossoms, 110–11
GLH, 208
goat testicles, 238, 241–42
goat urine, 217
Goddard, Jonathan, 229
Godfrey's Cordial, 62
goiters, 227
gold, 35–43
gold chloride, 37, 38, 40
Golden Ointment, 79
Goldsmith, Oliver, 15–16, 18
gonorrhea, 120, 218
Goodyear, Charles, 266
gout, 16, 47, 64, 229, 231, 278, 294, 298
Grafenburg Water Cure, 175
Graham, James, 280
Graham, Sylvester, 253
Grant, Ulysses S., 103–4
Granville, Joseph Mortimer, 248
Grape Cure, 326
Greatrakes, Valentine, 320–21
Gross's Neuralgia Pills, 28

H
Haglund, Daisy, 256
Hague International Opium Convention, 71
Haibel, Sophie, 130
halls of shame
    for antidotes, 124–26
    for cancer, 326–28
    for eye care, 324–25
    for men's health, 206–8

for weight loss, 266–68
for women's health, 56–58
Halsted, William Stewart, 100, 101
Hamilton, Alexander, 7, 62
hand washing, 190
hangings, 221–22
hangman's salve, 227
hangman's stroke, 222, 232
Hargraves, Fred, 41
Harrison Narcotics Act (1914), 71
hashish, 195
hatter's shakes, 6
Hauser, Gayelord, 324
Hawes, William, 90
hawk poop, 58
Haycraft, John Berry, 220
Hazzard, Linda, 255–57, 261, 265
headaches, 151–52, 158, 164, 185, 193, 214, 231, 237, 275
hearing loss, 213
heart, dried, 226
heart arrhythmias, 313
heart disease, 94, 108, 237
heart failure, 229
Heart of a Dog (Bulgakov), 241
Hell, Maximilian (Father Hell), 283, 284
Helmont, Jan Baptiste van, 222, 228
hemlock, 64, 195
hemochromatosis, 139
hemorrhages, 120, 131
hemorrhoids, 101, 134, 154, 169, 250–51
henbane, 195
Henry IV, 318
heparin, 243

hernias, 164
Herodotus, 17
heroic depletion therapy, 7, 135, 138, 219
heroin, 69–71
Hickman, Henry Hill, 196–97
Hicks, Thomas, 72–74
Hieronymus, T. Galen, 312
Hieronymus machine, 312
Hill, Mary, 52
Hippocrates, 17, 26–27, 57, 64, 118, 131, 142, 154, 156, 165, 168, 213, 222, 246, 326
hirudiculture, 219
hirudin, 213, 220
Hitler, Adolf, 81, 165
Hoffmann, Felix, 70
Hoffman's Drops, 204
Holmes, Oliver Wendell, 204
Homer, 64, 212
homicidality, 193
homosexual aversion therapy, 22
honeyed man, 226
hormone blockade, 328
horns, 125
horse, licking by, 320
hot flashes, 243
Huang Di Nei Jing texts, 134
Hughes, Bart, 142
Hui, King, 212
humoral theory, 5, 10, 17, 19, 131, 135, 139, 167, 213, 222
Hunt, Roland, 300
Hutchinson, Jonathan, 29–30
Huxley, Aldous, 324
hydrargyrum, 8–9
hydrogen gas, 199

hydropathic institutes,
175–78, 183, 295
hydropathy, 173–83
hydrophobia, 227
Hygienic Institute, 170, 172
hypertension, 47
hypnosis, 289–91
hypochondria, 6, 161
hypodermic syringe, 69
hypothermia, 112–13
hysterectomies, 57
hysteria, 6, 57, 161, 100,
212, 227, 245–50

I
Ibsen, Henrik, 103
ice-pick lobotomy, 148
Iliad (Homer), 212
Imaginary Invalid, The
(Molière), 167
impotence, 238–42, 275
infertility, 57
inflammation, 161
Influence of the Blue Ray of the
Sunlight and of the Blue
Colour of the Sky, The
(Pleasanton), 294
influenza, 4, 79
inheritance powder, 26
Innocent VIII, Pope, 224
insane asylums, 179–80
insanity, 134–35, 237–38
insomnia, 64, 199
insulin, 243
iodine, 268
ipecac (ipecacuanha), 22
iridology, 325

J
J. B. L. Cascade, 170, 172
Jacobs, Sarah, 259–60
jalap, 12
James, Robert, 16
James I, 88

Jamison, Alcinous Burton,
169
Jane Eyre (Bronte), 166
jaundice, 231, 302
Jayne's Carminative Balsam,
62
Jefferson, Thomas, 7
Jems, 79
Jenner, Edward, 236–37
jet lag, 302
Johnson, James Rawlins,
216–17
Johnson, Samuel, 308, 322
joint pain, 231
Jones, Stan, 42
Joyful News Out of the
New Found World
(Monardes), 85
Julius Caesar, 17
Julius Caesar (Shakespeare),
247
juniper berries, 106, 108–11

K
Kämpf, Johann, 166
Keeley, Leslie E., 36, 40–42
Keener Vision without Glasses
(Hauser), 324
Kellogg, John Harvey, 194,
253, 296, 298
Kennedy, Joe, 141
Kennedy, Rosemary,
140–41, 146, 148
kidneys, 120, 193
king's drops, 229
king's evil and king's touch,
314–28
Klaus, Frank, 241
Koch, Robert, 138
kohl, 21
Koller, Karl, 100
Kolletschka, Jakob, 190
Kratzenstein, Christian
Gottlieb, 274

L
laetrile, 327–28
lameness, 275
lancet, 132
Lane, Eugene, 35–36, 41
Lane, William, 327
Lane, William Arbuthnot,
193
lanolin, 243
Larrey, Jean, 188
Larsen, Kate Clifford, 148
laryngitis, 161
laudanum, 65–67
laughing gas, 199–202
leeches, 211–20, 237, 326
Leo XIII, Pope, 103
lethargy, 214
Letheon, 203–4
leucotome, 146, 148
leucotomy, 145–46
Lewis, Meriwether, 12
Leyden jars, 273
Li Shizhen, 226
Lidwina, Saint, 258–59
Life and Adventures of the
American Cowboy, The
(Stanley), 234
light, 292–302
light baths, 295, 296
Light Therapeutics (Kellogg),
296, 298
lightbulbs, 296
Lincoln, Abraham, 9
Linnaeus, Carl, 87
Lister, Joseph, 190
Liston, Robert, 188–89
lithotomy, 191
Little House on the Prairie
(Ingalls), 166
liver, 226
Lloyd's Cocaine Toothache
Drops, 101
lobotomy, 140–50
London Purple, 33

Long, Crawford, 204
Longfellow, Henry
    Wadsworth, 308
Louis, Pierre, 219–20
Louis IX, 321–22
Louis XIV, 19, 168–69, 319,
    323
Louis XV, 319
lovesickness, 134, 159
Lupercalia, 247
lupus, 296
Lytta vesicatoria, 159–60

M
Macbeth (Shakespeare),
    317
MacElhone, Harry, 241
Macfadden, Bernarr, 261,
    265
Macklis, Roger, 54
MacLeod, John, 46
mad hatter's disease, 6
Madame Bovary (Flaubert),
    277
madness, 143
maggots, 237
magnetic healing practice,
    286
magnetized water, 282
malaise, 158
malaria, 28, 166, 168, 169
malnourishment, 257–60
malpractice suits, 191
mandrake, 195
mania, 38, 134–35
man's grease, 227
Mantegazza, Paolo, 99–100
Marconi, Guglielmo, 304
Mariani, Angelo, 102–3
Marie Antoinette, 135, 288
Marx, Karl, 29
Marx Brothers, 241
Mary, Queen of Scots, 125
Master Cleanse, 262

masturbation, 194, 207, 245,
    253, 277. *see also* sex
Mayer, Nathan, 69
McCormick, Harold Fowler,
    240
Melampus, 245–46
melancholy, 4, 134–35, 143,
    159
mellified man, 226
men's health, 206–8
menstrual afflictions, 214,
    216
mental illness, 145
menthol, 162
mercurial erethism, 6, 9, 13
mercuric chloride, 10
mercurons chloride, 5
mercury, 3–14, 116
Mesmer, Franz Friedrich
    Anton, 281–86, 288–89,
    290
mesmerism, 287
metabolism, boosts to, 266,
    268
Metatone, 81
methyl salicylate, 162
miasmas, 166, 170
midazolam, 205
migraines, 231
Millennium Oxygen
    Cooler, 182
mineral water, 182
mirrors, 325
misplaced organs, 193
Mithridates VI, 125
Molière, 167
Monardes, Nicolás, 85
Moniz, Egas, 145
Monkey Gland Cocktail,
    241
monkey gland surgery,
    240–41
monoclonal antibodies, 328
Morell, Theodor, 81

Morgan, Thomas Hunt, 236
morning sickness, 29
morphine, 62, 68–69, 96, 101
Morton, William, 202–4
mouth-to-mouth rescue
    breathing, 90
Mozart, Wolfgang
    Amadeus, 129–30
Mrs. Moffat's Shoo-Fly
    Powders for
    Drunkenness, 23
Mrs. Winslow's Soothing
    Syrup, 62, 71
mucous colitis, 298
multiple sclerosis, 259
mummies and mumia, 65,
    229–31
Munchausen syndrome, 194
muscle stimulators, 208
mustard gas, 99
My Lobotomy (Dully), 150
mysterious powers
    animal magnetism, 281–91
    electricity, 271–80
    king's touch, 314–28
    light, 292–302
    radionics, 303–13

N
N-acetylcysteine (NAC), 126
Napoleon, 33
Narcan, 71
Natural Hygiene
    movement, 260–61, 263
Nature Cure, 261, 263
neosalvarsan, 33
nepenthe, 64
nephropexy, 193
nephroptosis, 193
Nero, 27, 126
nerve blocks, 205
nervous exhaustion, 182
nervous fits, 229
neurasthenia, 79

New Concepts in Diagnosis and Treatment (Abrams), 304
Nicot, Jean, 85, 87
nicotine, 85, 92
Niemann, Albert, 99
night air, 166
nitrous oxide, 199–202
No-Breakfast Plan, The (Dewey), 260–61
nose writing, 324
nosebleeds, 229
novocaine, 205
nursing mothers/wet nurses, 29, 63, 109
Nuxated Iron, 206

O
obesity, 164, 296
Oesterlin, Franziska, 284–85
oil of human fat, 227
opiates, 36, 61–71, 96, 161
opioids, 205
opium, 62, 63–65, 71, 195, 325
Oporinus, Johannes, 65
organ disease, 212
organ donation and transplantation, 232
orgone and orgone boxes, 251–54
Osborne, Dr., 214, 216
Oscilloclast, 308–10
Osler, William, 60
ox brain, 238
oxygenated water, 182–83

P
pacemakers, 279
paclitaxel, 328
Paganini, Niccolò, 13
Paracelsus, 5, 10, 18, 34, 38, 65, 222, 230, 257, 284

Paradis, Maria Theresia von, 286
paralysis, 76–77, 169–70, 274, 294
parasites, 4, 5, 28, 225
Paré, Ambroise, 125, 154, 156–58, 231
Parkinson's disease, 22
Pasteur, Louis, 138, 190
patent medicines, viii, 28, 101
Patin, Guy, 19
Patterson, Mary, 287
Pavlov, Ivan, 236
pearls, 125–26
peas, 160
Peczely, Ignaz von, 325
pelvic douche, 180
pelvic massages, 247–48
Pemberton, John, 96, 104
penicillin, 34
penis rings, 207
penises, 206–7, 277
Pepys, Samuel, 308, 315
performance-enhancing drugs. *see* strychnine
periwinkle, 328
perpetual pills, 20–21
Phelps, Michael, 139
Philip I, 315
Philip Morris, 93
Philumenus, 22
phlebotomy instruments, 137
phlyctenotherapy, 161
Pidoux, Doctor, 78
piles. *see* hemorrhoids
pills, gilded, 38
Pink's Disease, 4
Pius X, Pope, 103
plague, 19, 66, 91, 109, 119, 124, 166, 231, 237, 274, 300
Plain Facts for Old and Young (Kellogg), 253

plants & soil
    alcohol, 105–14
    cocaine, 95–104
    earth, 115–26
    opiates, 61–71
    strychnine, 72–82
    tobacco, 83–94
Pleasanton, Augustus J., 292–95
Pliny the Elder, 22, 57–58, 108, 125, 223, 225
Pneumatic Institution for Relieving Disease by Medical Airs, 199–200
pneumonia, 139
Poe, Edgar Allan, 308
poisons, 116, 120, 124–26, 231
polyeythemia vera, 139
poor sinner's fat, 227
poppies, 63–64
Power, Tyrone, 313
Poyen, Charles, 287
pregnancy, 29, 121, 227. *see also* childbirth
Premarin, 243
Priessnitz, Vincent, 173–75
Primitive Physick, 88
Professor Modevi's Beard Generator, 208
Prohibition, 114
propofol, 205
prostate gland warmer, 207
psoriasis, 28, 302
psychosurgery, 145, 150
ptomaines, 166–67, 171
pucula emetic, 20
Pulvermacher, 276–77
Pure Food and Drug Act (1906), viii, 47, 236, 325
pyridine, 91
Pythagoras, 257

Q
Qin Shi Huang, 8
quicksilver, 8–9
Quimby, Phineas Parkhurst, 287

R
R. J. Reynolds Tobacco Company, 94
rabies, 157, 227
radiation treatment, 54, 328
Radiendocrinator, 49–50
Radioclast, 306–7
radionics, 303–13
Radithor, 45, 52–53, 54
radium, 44–58
Radium Spa Hotel, 55
radon, 47–58
Ramazzini, 138
ratsbane eaters, 30–31
reconstructive surgeries, 220
rectal dilators, 250–51
Recto Rotor, 208
red coloring, 243
red nitre, 57
redheads, 225
Reich, Wilhelm, 251–52, 254
respiratory infections, 202
Revigator, 48
rheumatism, 47, 274, 278, 283
rheumatoid arthritis, 43
Rife, Royal Raymond, 327
Rife Frequency Generator, 327
ringworm, 231
Rod of Asclepius, 14
Roger's Cocaine Pile Remedy, 101
roundworms, 289
Routh, Charles, 63

Ruppert, Jacob, 114
Rush, Benjamin, 6–7, 12, 23, 135, 138, 179, 328

S
Salerno, Trotula de, 246
salt, as emetic, 22
salvarsan, 33
Sandall, Leonard, 75
sanitation, 190, 192
scarificator, 132
scarlet fever, 296
scent treatments, 56–57
schizophrenia, 144
sciatica, 278
Scott, Dr., 275–76
scrofula, 314–23
scrotal tumors, 289
scurvy, 16, 202, 296
seasonal affective disorder, 302
seawater, 22
seizures, 170
Semmelweis, Ignaz, 190
Seneca the Younger, 17
sepsis, 190
Sertürner, Friedrich Wilhelm Adam, 68
seton, 160
Seven Keys to Colour Healing, The (Hunt), 300
sex, 78–79, 244–54. *see also* masturbation
sexual dysfunction, 164, 206–7, 238–42
Shakespeare, William, 247, 317
shark cartilage, 327
Sharks Don't Get Cancer (Lane and Comac), 327
Shelton, Herbert, 261, 263–64
Shields, Alexander, 320
silver, 42

Simpson, James Young, 197–98
Sinclair, Upton, 265, 310–12
skin, 225, 227
skull moss, 229
skulls, 228–29
sleep apnea, 194
sleeping sickness, 28, 34
smallpox, 91, 236–37
smelling salts, 57
Smith, Elizabeth, 177
smoking, 83–84, 92–94
snails, 237
snake oil, 233–36
snakebites, 231
Snodgrass, J. E., 132
snuff, 87
Societies of Harmony, 288
Sollmann, Torald, 29
soporific sponge, 195
Soranus, 246
Spanish fly, 159–60
spanking, 247
Spectro-Chromo, 299–301
sperm donation, 232
sperm whales, 237
spiderwebs, 237
spinal curvature, 291
spondylotherapy, 304
spray-on hair, 208
St. Bernard dogs, 112
St. Hubert's key, 157
St. James's Fever Powder, 16
St. Vitus Dance disease, 38
Stanley, Clark, 233–34, 236
Stanton, Elizabeth Cady, 177
Starvation Heights, 256–57, 261
static electricity, 273
stem cells, 232
Stevenson, Robert Louis, 102, 103
stibnite, 21, 23

stomach ailments, 214
stress, 182
Striga, 119, 120–21
Stringer self-treating device, 207
strokes, 192–93
strychnine, 72–82, 206
stuttering, 192, 321
suicidality, 193
sunbathing, 264
suppository medicine, 171
surgery, 127, 191–94
Surgical Ray, 300
surrogacy, 232
Sushruta Samhita, 135, 192, 213–14
Swatsenburg, Lee, 262
sweating, 266, 298
swelling, 229
swooning, 229
Sydenham, Thomas, 66
syphilis, 4, 10–13, 19, 28, 33–34, 40, 231, 308

T
tapeworms, 266
tartar emetic, 20, 23, 161
Tasteless Ague and Fever Drops, 28
Taylor, Edward, 226, 227
Temple of Health, 280
terra sigillata, 115–17, 119–22
Tesla, Nikola, 301
testicles, 13, 58, 218, 237, 238–42
Thatcher, Margaret, 279
Therapeutic and Electrical Institute, 278
therapeutic fasting movement, 260–61
theriac, 126
Thermalaid, 207
Thölde, Johann, 19, 20

Thomas, R. W., 48
Thompson, Isaac, 325
Thorazine, 150
Thumblardt, Wendel, 115–17
Thurneysser zum Thurn, Leonhard, 39
thyroid, 227, 266, 268
Tiberius, 27
tobacco, 83–94
tonsillitis, 194
tonsils and tonsillectomies, 194, 211–12
tonsures, 133
tools
    anesthesia, 195–208
    blistering, 151–62
    bloodletting, 129–39
    cautery, 151–62
    clysters, 163–72
    cold water cure, 173–83
    enemas, 163–72
    hydropathy, 173–83
    lobotomy, 140–50
    surgery, 184–94
toothpaste, 49, 92
toxiphagi, 30–31
Trall, Russell, 247
traumatic brain injury, 142
treacle, 126
Treatise on the Medicinal Leech (Johnson), 216–17
Trepanation: The Cure for Psychosis (Hughes), 142
trepanning, 142, 143
trephine, 144
Treponema pallidum, 10
triboelectric effect, 273
Trosseau, Doctor, 78
Trota, 58, 246
Trotula, 58
Trout, Jennie Kidd, 278
Tschudi, Johann Jakob von, 30

tuberculosis, 47, 70, 79, 164, 199, 212, 315
tumors, 230, 313
typhoid fever, 169, 296
typhus, 166
Tyrrell, Charles A., 169–70, 172
Tyson, Stuart, 14

U
ulceration, 120
ulcers, 230–31
unicorn horns, 125
urinary problems, 193
urine, 217, 243

V
vaccinations, 236–37
Valentine, Basil, 18–19, 20
Vanhove, M., 77
varicose veins, 313
venereal disease, 212.
    see also gonorrhea;
    syphilis
Verne, Jules, 103
vertigo, 214
vesicants, 161
vibrators, 248–50
Victoria, Queen, 103
Vigo, Giovanni da, 156
Vin Mariani, 103–4
vinca alkaloids, 328
violet ray, 301
Virgil, 247
Vita Radium, 50
vitamin B-17, 327–28
Volstead Act (1919), 114
Volta, Alessandro, 273
Voltaire, 10, 323
vomiting, 16–18, 199
Von Schilling Surgical Ray, 300
Voronoff, Serge, 238–39, 240–41

W

Wakley, Thomas, 191
wallpaper, arsenic in, 33
wandering uterus, 56, 246
Ward, Joshua, 21
Ward's Drop and Ward's
    Pill, 21
Warren, John Collins, 200,
    202–3
warts, 222
Washington, George, 136,
    138
water cure, cold, 173–83
Watts, James, 146, 148, 149
weasel testicles, 58
Wei Boyang, 37
weight loss, 266–68, 275
Wells, Horace, 200, 202
wens, 222, 232
werewolfism, 159

wet dress, 177–78
wet sheet, 176–77
wet-cupping, 139
White, James and Walter,
    221–22
Wilde, Oscar, 102, 308
Wilkinson, Mr., 216
William and Mary, 322
William the Conqueror,
    110
Williams, Charles, 161
Williamson, Claire, 256–57
Williamson, Dora, 256–57
wine, 96, 102–4, 106–8
Withals, John, 257
Wolfgang II, 116–17
women's health, 50, 56–58,
    64, 180, 204, 214,
    216, 245–46. *see also*
    childbirth; pregnancy

wonder foods, 324
Wood, Alexander, 69
Woodley, Shailene, 123
Worm Lozenges, 79
Worth, William, 109
wound care, 237
Wright, Charles Romley
    Adler, 69

Y

yellow fever, 7
yew trees, 328
Yonge, James, 154
*Your Body's Many Cries for
    Water* (Batmanghelidj),
    181

Z

zootherapy, 236

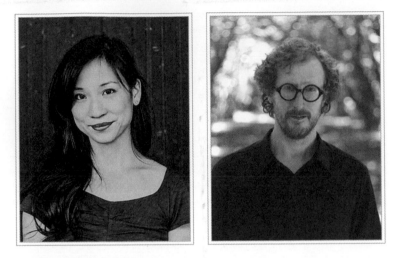

LYDIA KANG, MD, is a practicing internal medicine physician and author whose novels include *Control, Catalyst, The November Girl,* and *A Beautiful Poison.*

NATE PEDERSEN is a freelance journalist whose work appears in numerous publications including *The Guardian, The Believer,* and the *San Francisco Chronicle.*